**GLAND
P KEY**

OTHER BEST TENT CAMPING TITLES

Arizona
The Carolinas
Colorado
Florida
Georgia
Illinois
Kentucky
Maryland
Michigan
Minnesota
Missouri and the Ozarks
Montana
New Jersey
New Mexico
New York State
Northern California
Ohio
Oregon
Pennsylvania
The Southern Appalachian and Smoky Mountains
Southern California
Tennessee
Texas
Utah
Virginia
Washington
West Virginia
Wisconsin

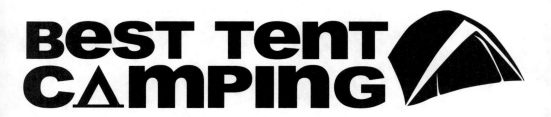

BEST TENT CAMPING

NEW ENGLAND

YOUR CAR-CAMPING GUIDE TO SCENIC BEAUTY, THE SOUNDS OF NATURE, AND AN ESCAPE FROM CIVILIZATION

Fourth Edition

LAFE LOW

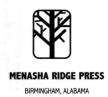

MENASHA RIDGE PRESS
BIRMINGHAM, ALABAMA

This book is for my son, Devin—my best camping buddy ever—
and for Douglas Low (1947–2008)
and Laurence W. Howard, Jr. (1931–2010).

Best Tent Camping: New England

Copyright © 2012 by Lafe Low
All rights reserved
Printed in the United States of America
Published by Menasha Ridge Press
Distributed by Publishers Group West
Fourth edition, first printing

Library of Congress Cataloging-in-Publication Data

Low, Lafe, 1962–
    Best tent camping. New England : Your car-camping guide to scenic beauty, the sounds of
nature, and an escape from civilization. / Lafe Low.—4th ed.
        p. cm.—(Best tent camping)
    ISBN 978-0-89732-964-4 (pbk.)—ISBN 0-89732-964-3 ()
        1. Camping—New England—Guidebooks. 2. Camp sites, facilities, etc.—
New England—Guidebooks. 3. Automobile travel—New England—Guidebooks.
    4. New England—Guidebooks. I. Title.
        GV191.42.N3L69 2012
        917.4—dc23

                                        2012012945

Editor: Ritchey Halphen
Cover design: Scott McGrew
Cover photos: All, iStockphoto.com—(front) Denis J. Tangney;
    (back, left–right) Denis J. Tangney, Frank van den Bergh, andipantz
Text design: Ian Szymkowiak/Palace Press International, Inc.
Cartography: Steve Jones, Lafe Low, and Scott McGrew
Indexing: Rich Carlson

Menasha Ridge Press
P.O. Box 43673
Birmingham, Alabama 35243
menasharidge.com

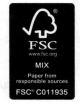

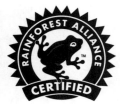

TABLE OF CONTENTS

ACKNOWLEDGMENTS

WHILE I WROTE THE WORDS and drove the miles in preparing this book, I enjoyed the tremendous benefit of support and inspiration from many people. Most of all, I would like to thank my family and my parents (all three of them!), Linsey Low, the late Douglas Low, and Larry Howard, for their endless encouragement, understanding, love, and patience, especially as I dragged them around to these campgrounds.

To the innumerable state-park rangers and volunteers I chatted with at campgrounds all over New England, and to the friendly folks at the private campgrounds I visited: I tip my hat to you. I'll be back soon, when I can stay a few days and relax!

—*Lafe Low*

PREFACE

NEW ENGLAND IS A REMARKABLE REGION. Nowhere else in the United States are you simultaneously so close to an ocean, mountains, lakes, and rivers. Drive a few hours, and the landscape and scenery change as rapidly and dramatically as the weather.

I've lived in New England all my life, moving around and experiencing almost all of the six New England states. (Rhode Island is the only New England state whose license plate hasn't graced my vehicle at one point or another.)

I am also somewhat of a creature of habit. Over the years I've found spots where I can experience the solitude, wonder, and awesome beauty of the wilderness, and I keep going back to those same spots. There's a comfortable cloak of familiarity, but in cruising back to familiar territory, I've inadvertently blown by some incredible areas.

As I traversed New England to research this book, I discovered some magical spots I might never have found otherwise, and for that I am thankful. The beachfront solitude of Washburn Island, the isolation and deep wilderness beauty of Pillsbury State Park and Gilson Pond, the natural cathedral of site 21 at Branbury State Park—these are places that gave me chills when I first found them. Now I'll return to these spots for longer visits. When you get the chance to visit here, I hope you have an equally memorable experience.

Enjoy the ride.

INTRODUCTION

WELCOME TO THE FOURTH EDITION OF *Best Tent Camping: New England.* As in previous iterations of the book, I've removed five old campgrounds and added five new ones for this edition. With each new edition, the process of identifying five profiles to remove becomes much more difficult. Sometimes that's easy if a campground goes all-RV or completely shuts down. Most often, though, it's hard to pick out the campgrounds that are my least favorite of this group of 60.

Finding five new ones, on the other hand, is a delight. The research is the best part of the process! I think you'll enjoy the new campgrounds outlined in this fourth edition: Gilson Pond and Wildwood in New Hampshire, Shawme-Crowell in Massachusetts, and Hopeville Pond and Mashamoquet Brook in Connecticut.

New England has hundreds of campgrounds. Winnowing the list down to 60 was no easy task. The ones represented in this book are what I consider 60 of the greatest campgrounds in New England.

Plenty of wonderful campgrounds and campsites out there didn't make it into the book but are still well worth checking out. In developing the list of campgrounds to explore here, I took into account numerous factors, one of which was accessibility. I wanted to profile campgrounds that offer a peaceful wilderness experience and are also accessible enough for a quick escape.

Of course, there are some pristine, incredibly remote campsites carved out of the wilderness of northern Maine and northern New Hampshire, or tucked away on islands in several New England lakes that aren't included in this book—yet. They may be in future editions, so stay tuned.

One other thing you'll no doubt notice is that most of the campgrounds profiled here are either state-park or national-forest campgrounds. That's no accident, as they tend to provide more of a wilderness experience. I've come to realize it's probably a simple matter of economics. Many private campgrounds cater to the RV crowd because, quite frankly, those folks spend a lot more money when they visit. RV campers need hookups, which cost money, and they tend to stay for long periods of time.

In researching previous editions, I've come across private campgrounds that closed down for good because of economic hardship. I also had to remove a private campground that was featured in the first two editions after it went all-RV.

There are some notable exceptions, however. The Mount Desert Campground leaps to mind. While it neither excludes nor bends over backward to bring in the land yachts, the simple fact of its rugged, waterfront topography limits the size and quantity of RVs. Another exception: the Hermit Island Campground. Both Mount Desert and Hermit Island are fabulous spots that you should make time to discover. I hope you'll be able to visit many of the other campgrounds profiled in this book, and I hope you'll agree that they're among the region's best.

THE OVERVIEW MAP AND OVERVIEW-MAP KEY

Use the overview map on the inside front cover to determine the exact location of each campground. The campground's number appears not only on the overview map but also on the map key facing the overview map, in the table of contents, and on the profile's first page.

This book is organized by state, as indicated in the table of contents. A legend that explains the symbols found on the campground-layout maps appears on the inside back cover.

CAMPGROUND-LAYOUT MAPS

Each profile contains a detailed map that provides an overhead view of campsites, internal roads, facilities, and other key elements.

GPS COORDINATES

Backpackers and campers were the first group to adopt GPS technology. Now it seems everyone has a box squawking directions on their dashboard. As GPS tools have become more and more affordable, it makes plenty of sense to include that information in each chapter. This book provides each campground's entrance coordinates in latitude–longitude format.

THE CAMPGROUND PROFILE

In addition to maps, each profile contains a concise but informative narrative describing the campground and individual sites. This text is enhanced with four helpful sidebars: Ratings, Key Information, Getting There (accurate driving directions that lead you to the campground from the nearest major roadway), and GPS Coordinates (see above). On the first page of each profile is a Ratings box.

THE RATING SYSTEM

Each campground is rated from one to five in each of the following categories: beauty, privacy, spaciousness, quiet, security, and cleanliness. This was often a tough call, because each section within each campground might warrant different ratings. So the ratings you'll see at the beginning of each profile are representative of the campground as a whole. While you may see a three or four for privacy overall, you'll probably find a couple of sites tucked in the far reaches of the campground that clearly rate at least a five.

BEAUTY This factor may seem obvious but is often elusive or, at the very least, subjective. What appeals to one camper may not appeal to another. I prefer campgrounds and campsites set deep within the woods. The greater the sense of natural solitude a campsite provides, the better it is, at least in my view.

Speaking of views, many of the campgrounds profiled here, and certainly many of the individual sites within these campgrounds, are arrayed along the shores of a lake, a pond, or even the ocean. These campsites are off the charts when it comes to site beauty. If there were a six-star rating, sites like those situated along the waters of Moosehead Lake, Half Moon Pond, and Somes Sound would easily deserve it. Also, many sites at campgrounds close to the water provide dramatic water views even if they aren't right on shore. These sites, too, are among some of the most spectacularly scenic.

PRIVACY   When you set up your campsite, the last thing you want is to feel as if you're piled up on top of your neighbors. Even in campgrounds where the sites aren't huge, if they are encircled by a relatively dense forest and arranged with an eye toward privacy, you can find a site that puts you in your own slice of the woods.

SPACIOUSNESS   Some New England campsites are barely big enough for your tent, a picnic table, and a fire ring. Others are large enough to accommodate a house. I don't typically need a lot of room when I'm camping, but I don't want to pitch my tent right next to the picnic table. This rating will give you an idea of how much elbow room you can expect when you set up camp.

QUIET   This is another factor that is particularly important to me. I like campsites that are very well isolated—secluded from neighboring sites and the rest of the campground. So I find it especially distracting if I can hear a persistent drone of cars and trucks blasting by on a nearby road, the steady whine of powerboats zipping by on a lake, or (worse yet) the sounds of portable TVs and sound systems.

You can rest assured that I paid close attention to the noisiness of these campgrounds. In some cases, parts of a campground are close to a main road, while the rest of the campground is separated by enough distance and enough forest to block out road noise.

SECURITY   It's a shame that this even has to be a factor, but you have to be practical. I've never had anyone steal or rummage through my stuff at any of the campgrounds mentioned here, but there are some that feel safer to me than others. The size of the campground and its proximity to urban areas are the primary aspects I considered when making my security determinations. Be prudent, even when it looks as if there's no one around. It's not a bad idea to lock up your car and your bike when you retire to your tent for the night. A bit of precaution can go a long way toward making sure you return home with all your gear.

CLEANLINESS   Most of the campgrounds profiled here scored highly on the cleanliness scale. This is true for a couple of reasons. First, I think that most people who enjoy the idea of spending a night in the woods are also inclined to take good care of the forest and their campsites. Second, many state parks make extraordinary efforts to keep their campsites well maintained. When you see the park rangers or other staff about the campground, take a moment to say hi and thank them for keeping the campground clean.

Of course, all this depends on you doing your part as well. Even though campgrounds are heavily traveled and well-worn spots, do what you can to leave no trace. Pack out everything you packed in (and even a little more). Please don't pile your trash in the fireplace, and don't try to burn things that aren't supposed to burn or that emit dangerous fumes.

Even at the cleanest of campgrounds and campsites, whenever I find a stray piece of paper, a bottle cap, or a cigarette butt (especially the latter), I always take a moment to reach down and pick it up to dispose of it properly. If everyone is mindful to be as gentle with the forest as possible, it will remain pristine for generations to come. Every time you pick up a bit of trash in the woods, consider it doing a favor for your children or grandchildren, even if you don't have any yet!

NEW ENGLAND WEATHER

Even during the summer, it's prudent to pack a fleece jacket and a waterproof jacket. It seems that on at least half of the occasions where I find myself camping outside, it rains. I think the camping gods start chuckling every time they see me grab my tent.

Anyway, it's a good idea to be prepared for any kind of weather. That doesn't mean bring your snowshoes in August, but by all means bring a warm jacket and something water-resistant. The weather in New England can and does change faster than the scenery as you drive from Cape Cod to the Berkshires. Have something warm, have something dry. You'll be much more comfortable and safer.

Also, even if it's been a bright, sunny day, foul weather can blow in at any time, and frequently does. I've been tempted on many nights to ignore the rainfly on my tent and just leave it in the car. This can be a bad idea, especially if it starts raining at 2 a.m. Be ready and you'll be happy.

CANOE AND KAYAK CAMPING

Several of the campgrounds profiled here are accessible only by canoe or kayak. While this poses a number of logistical and packing challenges, the rewards of absolute solitude and camping right on the water are well worth the extra effort.

You need to consider a few important safety factors when canoe- or kayak-camping. First and foremost, you must be comfortable with your paddling skills before you add the weight of camping gear to your boat. Don't plan a camping trip on your first attempt at paddling a canoe or kayak.

With a sea kayak, try to stow all your gear in the sealed bulkheads. It may be tempting to strap your tent or sleeping pad to the deck, but anything protruding above deck level will make your kayak less stable. Besides catching the wind, it also raises the boat's center of gravity. Keep all your gear below decks.

Most touring kayaks have fore and aft storage compartments. Try to spread your gear between them evenly—even if all your gear will fit in the aft compartment—to ensure that your kayak floats level. Once you've packed your boat, take it for a test float. Get it into water deep enough that it floats freely. If it looks like you're popping a wheelie or about to take a nosedive, or if you're listing to one side, you need to redistribute your gear. Keep these same principles in mind when stowing gear in a canoe: try to balance the load in the center, and distribute it evenly fore and aft.

All that said, you can pack an amazing amount of gear in a canoe or kayak. Before I packed for my first-ever group trip, we divided the group gear. I stowed the latter in my aft compartment and my personal stuff in the forward compartment—there was still plenty of room in each.

You can do a few things to make your canoe- or kayak-camping trip more convenient. For your first dinner at your island campsite, prepare something in advance, freeze it in a Tupperware container, and then when dinnertime arrives, all you have to do is heat it up and you're ready to eat. Also, you should wrap tightly in a large plastic garbage bag any gear that you haven't stored in a dry bag. Anything you store in the bulkheads or open in your canoe can and most likely will get wet. There's nothing worse than reaching for a jacket or vest to wear, only to find it damp or soggy.

THE CAMPFIRE AWAITS

There's nothing like a night spent outside. The soft crackle of a campfire, the flickering light thrown about the forest, the satisfaction of the day's travels, and the anticipation of tomorrow's adventures—it's a potent combination.

The camping tips here and the descriptions of the campgrounds that follow will steer you to a memorable experience. I've profiled campgrounds from the farthest northern reaches of Vermont, New Hampshire, and Maine to the seashores of Connecticut and Rhode Island, and everything in between. Some are familiar haunts, some are unexpected hidden gems; all are spectacular.

Wherever you choose to go camping in New England—from the sandy bluffs of Nickerson State Park to the deep woods of Clarksburg State Forest, from the absolute solitude of Warren Island to the cool, crisp mountain air of Crawford Notch Campground—you're in for a memorable and magical trip.

FIRST-AID KIT

A useful first-aid kit may contain more items than you might think necessary. These are just the basics. Prepackaged kits in waterproof bags are available (Atwater Carey and Adventure Medical make them). As a preventive measure, take along sunscreen and insect repellent. Even though quite a few items are listed here, they pack down into a small space:

Ace bandages or Spenco joint wraps

Adhesive bandages

Antibiotic ointment (Neosporin or the generic equivalent)

Antiseptic or disinfectant, such as Betadine or hydrogen peroxide

Aspirin or acetaminophen

Benadryl or the generic equivalent, diphenhydramine (in case of allergic reactions)

Butterfly-closure bandages

Epinephrine in a prefilled syringe (for people known to have severe allergic reactions to such things as bee stings)

Gauze (one roll)

Gauze compresses (six 4 x 4–inch pads)

Matches or pocket lighter

Moleskin or Spenco 2nd Skin

Waterproof first-aid tape

Whistle (it's more effective in signaling rescuers than your voice is)

ANIMAL AND PLANT HAZARDS

Ticks

Ticks are often found on brush and tall grass, waiting to hitch a ride on a warm-blooded passerby. Among the local varieties of ticks, the nymph deer tick is the primary carrier of Lyme disease. You can use several strategies to reduce your chances of ticks getting under your skin. Some people choose to wear light-colored clothing, so ticks can be spotted before they make it to the skin. Most important, be sure to visually check your hair, the back of your neck, your armpits, and your socks at the end of the hike. During your posthike shower, take a moment to do a more complete body check. For ticks that are already embedded, removal with tweezers is best. Use disinfectant solution on the wound.

Poison Ivy, Oak, and Sumac

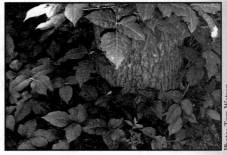

Poison ivy *(right)* occurs as a vine or ground cover, 3 leaflets to a leaf; poison oak occurs as either a vine or shrub, also with 3 leaflets; and poison sumac flourishes in swampland, each leaf having 7 to 13 leaflets. Urushiol, the oil in the sap of these plants, is responsible for the rash. Within 14 hours of exposure, raised lines and/or blisters will appear on the affected area, accompanied by a terrible itch. Refrain from scratching, because bacteria under your finger-nails can cause an infection. Wash and dry the rash thoroughly, applying calamine lotion to help dry out the rash. If itching or blistering is severe, seek medical attention. If you do come into contact with one of these plants, remember that oil-contaminated clothes, pets, or hiking gear can easily cause a rash on you or someone else, so wash not only any exposed parts of your body but also clothes, gear, and pets, if applicable.

Photo: Tom Watson

TIPS FOR A HAPPY CAMPING TRIP

There's nothing worse than a bad camping trip, especially because it's so easy to have a great one. Here are some pointers for making your outing a happy one.

- **RESERVE YOUR SITE AHEAD OF TIME,** especially if it's a weekend or holiday, or if the campground is wildly popular. Many prime campgrounds require at least a six-month lead time on reservations. Check before you go.

- **PICK YOUR CAMPING BUDDIES WISELY.** A family trip is pretty straightforward, but you may want to reconsider inviting any grumpy friends or relatives who don't like bugs, sunshine, or marshmallows. After you know who's going, make sure everyone is on the same page regarding expectations of difficulty (amenities or the lack thereof, physical exertion, and so on), sleeping arrangements, and food preferences/requirements.

- **DON'T DUPLICATE EQUIPMENT** such as cooking pots and lanterns among campers in your party. Carry what you need to have a good time, but don't turn the trip into a major moving experience.

- **DRESS FOR THE SEASON.** Educate yourself on the temperature highs and lows of the specific area you plan to visit. It may be warm at night in the summer in your backyard, but up in the mountains it can be quite chilly.

- **PITCH YOUR TENT ON A LEVEL SURFACE,** preferably one covered with leaves, pine straw, or grass. Use a tarp or specially designed footprint to thwart ground moisture and to protect the tent floor. Do a little site maintenance, such as picking up the small rocks and sticks that can damage your tent floor and make sleep uncomfortable. If you have a separate tent rainfly but don't think you'll need it, keep it rolled at the base of the tent in case it starts raining at midnight.

- **IF YOU'RE UNCOMFORTABLE SLEEPING ON THE GROUND,** take a sleeping pad with you that is full-length and thicker than you think you might need. This will not only keep your hips from aching on hard ground, it will also help keep you warm. A wide range of thin, light, inflatable pads is available at camping stores; these are a much better choice than air mattresses, which conduct heat away from the body and tend to deflate during the night.

- **IF YOU'RE NOT HIKING IN TO A PRIMITIVE CAMPSITE,** there's no real need to skimp on food because of weight. Plan tasty meals and bring everything you will need to prepare, cook, eat, and clean up.

- **IF YOU TEND TO USE THE BATHROOM MULTIPLE TIMES AT NIGHT,** you should plan ahead. Leaving a warm sleeping bag and stumbling around in the dark to find the restroom—be it a pit toilet, a fully plumbed comfort station, or just the woods—is no fun. Keep a flashlight and any other accoutrements you may need by the tent door, and know exactly where to head in the dark.

- **STANDING DEAD TREES AND STORM-DAMAGED LIVING TREES** can pose a real hazard to tent campers. These trees may have loose or broken limbs that could fall at any time. When choosing a campsite or even just a spot to rest during a hike, look up.

CAMPING ETIQUETTE

Camping experiences can vary wildly depending on a variety of factors, such as weather, preparedness, fellow campers, and time of year. Here are a few tips on how to create good vibes with fellow campers and any wildlife you encounter.

- **OBTAIN ALL PERMITS AND AUTHORIZATION AS REQUIRED.** Make sure you check in, pay your fee, and mark your site as directed. Don't make the mistake of grabbing a seemingly empty site that looks more appealing than yours—it could be reserved. If you're unhappy with the site you've selected, check with the campground host for other options.

- **LEAVE ONLY FOOTPRINTS.** Be sensitive to the ground beneath you. Be sure to place all garbage in designated receptacles or pack it out if none are available. No one likes to see the trash someone else has left behind.

- **NEVER SPOOK ANIMALS.** It's common for animals to wander through campsites, where they may be accustomed to the presence of humans (and our food). An unannounced approach, a sudden movement, or a loud noise can startle them. Surprised animals can be dangerous to you, to others, and to themselves. Give them plenty of space.

- **PLAN AHEAD.** Know your equipment, your ability, and the area where you are camping—and prepare accordingly. Be self-sufficient at all times; carry necessary supplies for changes in weather or other conditions. A well-executed trip is a satisfaction to you and to others.

- **BE COURTEOUS TO OTHER CAMPERS,** hikers, bikers, and others you encounter. If you run into the owner of a large RV, don't panic. Just wave, feign eye contact, then walk slowly away.

- **STRICTLY FOLLOW THE CAMPGROUND'S RULES** regarding the building of fires. Never burn trash. Trash smoke smells horrible, and debris left in a fire pit or grill is unsightly.

VENTURING AWAY FROM THE CAMPGROUND

If you go for a hike, bike, or other excursion into the wilderness, here are some tips:

- **ALWAYS CARRY FOOD AND WATER,** whether you're planning to go overnight or not. Food will give you energy, help keep you warm, and sustain you in an emergency. Bring potable water, or treat lake or stream water by boiling or filtering it before you drink it.

- **STAY ON DESIGNATED TRAILS.** Most hikers get lost when they leave the trail. Even on the most clearly marked trails, there is usually a point where you have to stop and consider in which direction to head. If you become disoriented, don't panic. As soon as you think you may be off-track, stop, assess your current direction, and then retrace your steps to the point where you went astray. If you have absolutely no idea how to continue, return to the trailhead the way you came in. Should you become completely lost and have no idea how to return to the trailhead, remaining in place along the trail and waiting for help is most often the best option for adults, and always the best option for children.

- **BE ESPECIALLY CAREFUL WHEN CROSSING STREAMS.** Whether you're fording the stream or crossing on a log, make every step count. If you have any doubt about maintaining your balance on a log, go ahead and ford the stream instead. When fording a stream, use a trekking pole or stout stick for balance and face upstream as you cross. If a stream seems too deep to ford, turn back. Whatever is on the other side is not worth risking your life for.

- **BE CAREFUL AT OVERLOOKS.** Although these areas may provide spectacular views, they are potentially hazardous. Stay back from the edge of outcrops and be absolutely sure of your footing: a misstep can mean a nasty and possibly fatal fall.

- **KNOW THE SYMPTOMS OF HYPOTHERMIA.** Shivering and forgetfulness are the two most common indicators of this insidious killer. Hypothermia can occur at any elevation, even in the summer. Wearing cotton clothing puts you especially at risk because cotton, when wet, wicks heat away from the body. To prevent hypothermia, dress in layers using synthetic clothing for insulation, use a cap and gloves to reduce heat loss, and protect yourself with waterproof, breathable outerwear. If symptoms arise, get the victim to shelter, a fire, hot liquids, and dry clothes or a dry sleeping bag.

- **LIKEWISE, KNOW THE SYMPTOMS OF HEAT EXHAUSTION.** Excessive sweating, faintness or dizziness, clammy skin, vomiting, and paleness are all common symptoms. If symptoms arise, remove extra clothing, move to the shade, and drink plenty of water.

- **TAKE ALONG YOUR BRAIN.** Think before you act. Watch your step. Plan ahead. Avoiding accidents before they happen is the best strategy for a rewarding and relaxing hike.

GET OUT AND GET ACTIVE WITH THE APPALACHIAN MOUNTAIN CLUB
outdoors.org

WITH THE AMC, you can participate in a wide variety of outdoor activities, connect with new people, and help to protect the natural world you love. Join us and each year you'll receive a full year of our member magazine, *AMC Outdoors,* which will keep you informed of environmental issues and outdoor recreation opportunities—including hiking, paddling, biking, and snowshoeing—across the Appalachian region. You'll receive discounts on AMC's guided adventures, courses, lodging, and books. You can also join our Conservation Action Network to help increase public influence regarding critical conservation issues today at **outdoors.org/conservation/action.**

LEARN SOMETHING NEW: AMC Outdoor Adventures

DEVELOP YOUR OUTDOOR SKILLS and knowledge through AMC's outdoor-adventures program. Learn to rock-climb, snowshoe, or navigate by map and compass. From beginner backpacking and family canoeing to guided camping trips, you'll find something for any age or interest at spectacular locations throughout the Appalachian region, including the Maine Woods, White Mountains, Adirondacks, Catskills, and Delaware Water Gap. For a full listing and to sign up, go to **outdoors.org/recreation.**

BE OUR GUEST: AMC Destinations and Accommodations

FROM THE NORTH WOODS OF MAINE to the White Mountains to the Delaware Water Gap, AMC offers a wide variety of accommodations, from full-service lodges to backcountry huts, shelters, and campsites. Experience outdoor adventure at its best as our guest. Get trip suggestions, check lodging availability, and make reservations online at **outdoors.org/lodging.**

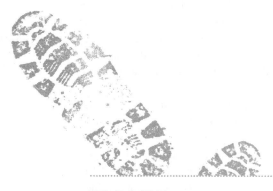

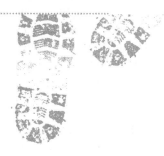

MAINE

1
BAXTER
STATE PARK

"**F**OREVER WILD"—**THOSE ARE THE WORDS** of Percival Baxter (1876–1969), a former governor of Maine, philanthropist, and conservationist who donated Mount Katahdin and the land surrounding it to the state, on the condition that it remain as he described it. "Forever wild" perfectly describes Baxter State Park as well. Its remoteness, size, and grandeur are profound. Baxter's intent was to keep the park undeveloped. Today, it's managed as a wildlife preserve first and as a recreation resource second.

At more than 200,000 acres, Baxter State Park is a huge place. There are actually 10 campgrounds within the park. Truth is, no matter where you end up in the park, you're bound to have a remote wilderness experience. Eight of the campgrounds you can reach by driving; the other two are hike-in areas. Camping in these areas requires a bit of additional effort, but the solitude and splendor are well worth it. If you're camping in Baxter State Park, by all means enjoy the convenience of the car-camping areas, but try to spend at least one night at Chimney Pond or Russell Pond, or even at one of the many truly remote wilderness campsites spread throughout the park.

After you enter the massive park through the Togue Pond Gate, along the park's southern border, you'll first come to is Abol Campground. It has 9 tent sites and 12 lean-tos; each lean-to can accommodate four people. Abol Campground sits at the trailhead for the Abol Trail, one of the routes to the summit of Katahdin, so this is one of several popular spots for hikers with designs on summiting the park's centerpiece peak.

Farther up Nesowadnehunk Tote Road, which encircles the perimeter of the park, is Katahdin Stream Campground, with 9 tent sites, 12 lean-tos that can fit 3 to 5 campers, and 3 group sites that can hold from 12 to 25. From here, hikers can head to the summit of Katahdin

> *A night spent camping in Baxter State Park, especially in one of the remote sites, is a true wilderness experience.*

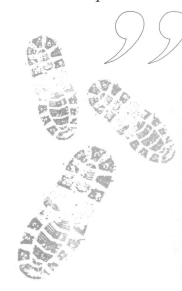

RATINGS

Beauty: ☆ ☆ ☆ ☆ ☆
Privacy: ☆ ☆ ☆ ☆
Spaciousness: ☆ ☆ ☆ ☆ ☆
Quiet: ☆ ☆ ☆ ☆ ☆
Security: ☆ ☆ ☆ ☆ ☆
Cleanliness: ☆ ☆ ☆ ☆

on the Hunt Trail, which is part of the Appalachian Trail. You can also easily get to the Owl Trail and the Grassy Pond Trail heading east.

Just to the southwest of Katahdin Stream you'll find Daicey Pond Campground. You get there by continuing north and west on Nesowadnehunk Tote Road, then heading south just before Foster Field Picnic Area. You could also hike there from Katahdin Stream Campground (or vice versa) on the Grassy Pond Trail. Daicey Pond Campground doesn't have any tent sites, but it does have 10 cabins with two to four beds each. The Appalachian Trail goes right through the campground. Another trail encircles Daicey Pond and leads to the short Lost Pond Trail, which takes you out to the still and secluded waters of its namesake.

Continuing northwest on Nesowadnehunk Tote Road along the western border of the park brings you to Nesowadnehunk Field Campground. Here you'll find 9 tent sites, 11 three- and four-person lean-tos, and 3 group sites. This campground has recently been restructured, so be sure to contact the rangers to make sure what you want is available. From here, you could easily get to the Doubletop Trail, a sturdy hike that takes you up and over Doubletop Mountain and offers some outrageous views of Katahdin.

Taking Roaring Brook Road off to the right from the Togue Pond gatehouse brings you first to Roaring Brook Campground. There are 10 tent sites (4 of which are walk-in sites), 9 lean-tos that accommodate anywhere from 2 to 6 people each, 3 group sites that hold up to 14, and a bunkhouse with room for 10. From here you have plenty of hiking options. Follow the Sandy Stream Pond Trail to the Turner Mountain Trail to hike up Turner Mountain. You could also head west on the Helon Taylor Trail to reach Katahdin.

KEY INFORMATION

ADDRESS: 64 Balsam Dr.
Millinocket, ME 04462

OPERATED BY: Maine Department of Conservation–Bureau of Parks and Lands

INFORMATION: 207-723-5140, baxterstateparkauthority.com

OPEN: May 15–Oct. 15, Dec. 1–March 31 (some campgrounds have variable dates)

SITES: 75 tent sites, 71 lean-tos, 5 bunkhouses, 13 group sites, and 22 cabins in 10 separate campgrounds

EACH SITE: Fire ring, picnic table (except hike-in sites)

ASSIGNMENT: Reservations strongly recommended; accepted Monday–Friday, 8 a.m.–4 p.m., otherwise first-come, first-served

REGISTRATION: At gatehouse and with ranger; check in after 1 p.m., check out by 11 a.m.

FACILITIES: Pit toilets, water spigots

PARKING: At sites

FEE: $14 nonresident vehicle fee to enter park; $30 for campground tent or lean-to site; $20 for backcountry tent or lean-to site; $11 per person, per night for bunkhouses; $55–$130 for cabins; $7 per person, per night for group sites ($42-per-night minimum)

RESTRICTIONS: *Pets:* Prohibited
Fires: Fire rings only
Alcohol: Prohibited
Vehicles: Parking at sites only

Head west on the Chimney Pond Trail from Roaring Brook Campground, and you'll come to Chimney Pond Campground. This is a remote and supremely beautiful spot. There are no tent sites here, but there are nine lean-tos that can each handle 4 people, and a bunkhouse that can fit 10. At least your tent is one less thing to carry.

Aside from being remarkably scenic, Chimney Pond Campground is a perfect base camp from which to summit Katahdin. You have your choice of the Saddle Trail, Cathedral Trail, or Dudley Trail. All of these hikes are steep and strenuous, so plan ahead and be prepared.

Also from the Roaring Brook Campground, follow the Russell Pond Trail to Russell Pond Campground, another incredibly remote and wild camping area. There are three tent sites, four lean-tos that can accommodate anywhere from four to eight people, and a bunkhouse for eight. This campground is also situated within a hub of trails, including the Russell Pond Trail and the Northwest Basin Trail (which leads to the North Peaks Trail) to the south, the Pogy Notch Trail to the north, and the Wassataquoik Lake Trail to the west. These are all fairly long hikes, so plan and pace yourself carefully, especially if you're doing a round-trip day hike from the campground. If you're looking for a shorter hike from Russell Pond Campground, try the Ledge Falls Trail, Grand Falls Trail, or Lookout Trail.

Entering the park from the northeast at Matagamon Gate Public Landing will get you close to the Trout Brook Farm and South Branch campgrounds. From the gatehouse, follow the road west to Trout Brook Farm Campground. This campground is primarily for tent campers, with 14 tent sites, four group sites for 8 to 14 people, and just one lean-to. From here, you can also hike in to a number of remote wilderness campsites. To the south, follow Five Ponds Trail to sites spread out along Littlefield Pond, Billfish Pond, and Long Pond. To the north, the lengthy, multiday Freezeout Trail brings you to remote campsites and lean-tos along Second Lake, Webster Brook, and Webster Lake.

From Trout Brook Campground, continue west on the road to The Crossing picnic area. Then head south on South Branch Road to find South Branch Campground, with 21 tent sites, 12 four-person lean-tos, and a bunkhouse for eight. This campground is at the northern tip of Lower South Branch Pond. From here, you can hike the short and sweet Ledges Trail or the Middle Fowler Trail.

There are also several excellent hikes to nearby peaks, including the North Traveler Trail, which leads up the mountain of the same name; the Howe Brook Trail, which follows its namesake brook past two dramatic waterfalls; and the Center Ridge Trail, which brings you to the summit of the Traveler. To the west of Upper and Lower South Branch ponds, the South Branch Mountain Trail takes you up and over Black Cat Mountain. These hikes aren't very long, but they are very steep. Never underestimate the intensity of the hiking anywhere within Baxter State Park.

Baxter State Park is a popular destination, with a finite number of campsites in and around the park. You could wing it by not making reservations, but you might end up disappointed or driving far out of your way to find an open site. If you do get jammed, there

MAP

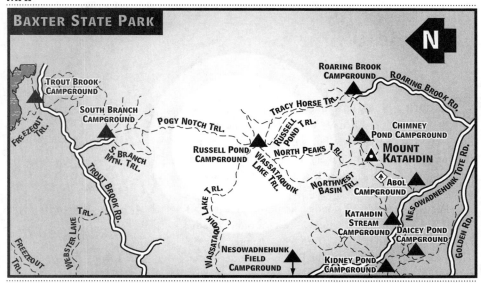

GETTING THERE

To get to the Togue Pond gatehouse, follow Baxter State Park Road northwest from the intersection of ME 11 and ME 157 in Millinocket. To get to the Matagamon Public Landing gatehouse from Patten, take US 1 north to ME 159 north to Grand Lake Road. Follow Grand Lake Road to the gatehouse.

are several private campgrounds just outside the park that provide a backup place to pitch your tent, but do yourself a favor and make a reservation. The peace of mind will be well worth it.

GPS COORDINATES

MATAGAMON PUBLIC LANDING
N46° 9.291887'
W68° 48.337269'

TOGUE POND GATEHOUSE
N45° 49.687600'
W68° 53.402345'

FOR SUCH A HUGE CAMPGROUND, most of the sites at Blackwoods still have a cozy atmosphere. The three-lane paved road (two lanes in, one out) accessing the campground might make you wonder what you're getting into, but rest assured, this is a great place to pitch a tent.

For one thing, Blackwoods Campground is just off Park Loop Road, which winds its way around Acadia National Park. Better still, from your campsite it's a short walk to the ocean, Sand Beach, Thunder Hole, Otter Cliff . . . the list goes on. The campground rests on the mostly flat forest floor beneath a loosely spaced forest canopy of mixed pine, balsam, hemlock, and hardwoods. The open forest lets lots of light filter through to the campground floor on sunny days, and a cool, nearly constant breeze blows in from the nearby Atlantic Ocean.

Blackwoods is separated into two main loops comprising 306 sites in all. There are also several group sites available by reservation only. The place is big! Blackwoods accepts reservations from May 1 to October 30. Making a reservation for an in-season trip is a wise idea, as Acadia National Park receives hordes of visitors during the summer and Blackwoods is likely to be full on most weekends.

Outside of those dates, it's first-come, first-served. About 50 campsites on Loop A are open year-round if you've come to Acadia to snowshoe or cross-country-ski on the massive network of carriage roads that wind their way in and around the park. I've frequently visited Blackwoods in the off-season. There has never been a fee, and I've always felt like I had the place to myself.

Looking at the sites within Loop A, you'll find several areas that are especially conducive to excellent tent camping. In the first subloop, sites 3, 4, 5, 7, and 10 through 19 are loosely spaced beneath a rich forest

> *This campground is set between the still of the forests and mountains of Acadia National Park and the thundering surf of the Atlantic Ocean.*

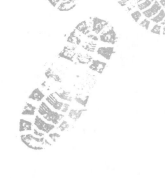

RATINGS

Beauty: ☆ ☆ ☆ ☆
Privacy: ☆ ☆ ☆
Spaciousness: ☆ ☆ ☆ ☆
Quiet: ☆ ☆ ☆ ☆
Security: ☆ ☆ ☆
Cleanliness: ☆ ☆ ☆ ☆

KEY INFORMATION

ADDRESS:	ME Route 3 Bar Harbor, ME 04609
OPERATED BY:	National Park Service
INFORMATION:	207-288-3338
OPEN:	Year-round; limited facilities Nov.–March
SITES:	306
EACH SITE:	Fire ring with grate, picnic table
ASSIGNMENT:	Reservations required May 1–Oct. 30, otherwise first-come, first-served
REGISTRATION:	Pay at ranger station at entrance to park; reservations: 877-444-6777, recreation.gov
FACILITIES:	Flush toilets, water spigots, showers and a camp store 0.5 mile away
PARKING:	1 vehicle per site, additional parking
FEE:	$10–$20 per site May 1–Oct. 30; $10 per site Nov. 1–March 31; park entrance pass required ($20 weekly, $40 annually)
RESTRICTIONS:	*Pets:* On leash or in cage at all times *Fires:* Fire rings only *Alcohol:* Sites only *Vehicles:* 1 per site *Other:* Quiet hours 10 p.m.–7 a.m.; check out by 10 a.m.

canopy. The sites have a welcoming blanket of pine needles, which makes a soft, aromatic bed for your tent and sleeping bag.

The next loop contains sites 2, 6, 8, 9, 22, 27, 29, 32, 33, and 34, which are also loosely spaced.

These two loops are quite close to the path leading down to the cliffs—a bonus. After the day crowds have cleared out, you've had your fireside dinner, and the campfire has died down, grab a flashlight and a mug of tea (or whatever suits your mood), and wander down the path and across Park Loop Road to watch the surf crash incessantly against the cliffs. That's a sight-and-sound combination of which I never tire.

Farther up the larger part of Loop A, the sites off to the left of the outer loop offer a nice sense of seclusion. Look for sites 104 through 108, 124 through 131, and 144 through 151. In truth, though, most of the sites within the sweeping expanse of Loop A will offer you a nice spot for your tent.

Over in Loop B, the sites are set apart from each other in several areas. The crossroad at the far end of this loop sets off sites 141, 143, 147, 150, 153, and 154. These are the sites I'd look for first in Loop B.

Taking the second or third left from the main outer loop will bring you to sites numbered in the high 60s and low 70s. Sites 65 through 73 have a good amount of elbow room between them. Site 45 is also stuck onto the far end of this loop. It's right on the main outer loop, but if you set up well within the site, you'll be fine.

There are also several group sites on the left side of Loop B. G4 and G5 offer the most space, although G5 is right across from the restrooms. Each of these reservation-only group sites has room for 15 to 20 campers. There's an amphitheater between Loop A and Loop B where rangers present evening slide shows and interpretive programs. Check the schedule at the campground entrance ranger station.

If you end up pitching your tent at the north end of Loop A, you'll be close to the South Ridge hiking trail, leading to the summit of Cadillac Mountain. Wherever you land at Blackwoods, or even if you stay elsewhere in or near Acadia National Park, a trip to the summit of Cadillac is one thing you won't want to miss. From the

MAP

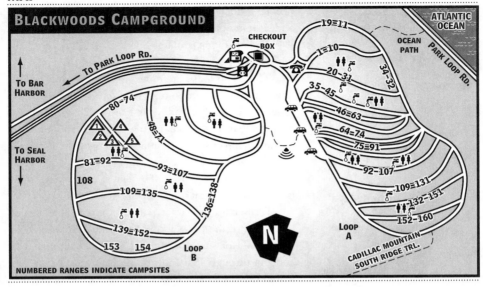

mountain, you'll have a sweeping, panoramic view that defies clichés and platitudes. Here's a tip: The sunsets are phenomenal, so much so that one per day may not be enough. Situate yourself along Park Loop Road to watch sunset. The instant it dips below the horizon, hop in your car and boogie up to the summit of Cadillac Mountain to watch it again!

GETTING THERE

From Ellsworth, follow ME 3 onto Mount Desert Island. Follow ME 3 to ME 102/198. Stay on ME 198 when it turns left, and follow this to ME 233. Follow ME 233 to the entrance to Acadia National Park, on the left. Enter the park and follow Park Loop Road to Blackwoods Campground, on the right.

GPS COORDINATES

N44° 18.612177'
W68° 12.232382'

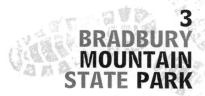

3
BRADBURY MOUNTAIN STATE PARK

> *The cool breezes and sunlight filtering through the trees add to the peaceful atmosphere of Bradbury Mountain State Park*

DESPITE ITS LOCATION, the campground at Bradbury Mountain State Park is exceptionally quiet. A bit of sporadic road noise emanates from ME 9, but the fragrant evergreen scent wafting through the loose forest is constant. There's an open, airy character to the forest that lets sunlight brighten the campground floor and the breezes blow through.

Pick your campsite and the ranger will come by to register you. Sites 3, 5, 6, 14, 15, 25, 28, 34, and 35 are first-come, first-served. You can reserve any of the other sites. A host site is on the right as you enter the campground, if you have any questions.

All of the sites have a hard, sandy surface that holds on to tent stakes. Sites 1 and 2 are moderately spacious. An old stone wall runs along the back of these sites. The open character of the forest here provides lots of light and nice breezes, but consequently not as much privacy as would a densely forested campground. Sites 8 and 9 are very spacious but open to each other and to the road. Sites 14 and 15 are very open to each other; they almost look like one extremely large, sandy spot. They would make a good pair of sites for a larger group or family needing two sites side-by-side. They're also designated as wheelchair-accessible.

The individual sites differ in size, as marked on the campground's map. The sites at Bradbury Mountain, however, are similar when it comes to their level of privacy. In general, the relatively light undergrowth affords only a mild sense of seclusion.

Three notable exceptions are sites 6, 12, and 16. These hike-in sites are reserved for tent campers only. The trail leading into 12 is next to site 11. It's about a 100-foot walk on a flat, sandy path to the site, which gives it a true wilderness feel.

The site itself is set within loosely spaced mixed forest with very little undergrowth. There's a very open,

RATINGS

Beauty: ✩ ✩ ✩ ✩
Privacy: ✩ ✩ ✩
Spaciousness: ✩ ✩ ✩ ✩
Quiet: ✩ ✩ ✩
Security: ✩ ✩ ✩ ✩
Cleanliness: ✩ ✩ ✩ ✩

breezy character to the forest here as well, but you're so separated from the rest of the campground that the sense of privacy is complete. From this site, you can look around 360 degrees, and all you'll see is the forest. Site 12 at Bradbury Mountain State Park offers a sense of seclusion equal to that of a backpacking site way off in the backcountry. Site 16 is another supremely secluded walk-in site. This site shares all the characteristics and accolades of site 12, but is actually a bit farther into the woods.

You might want to avoid sites 17 and 18, as these are right next to the shelter. Site 19 is huge but also has a very open feel. Exposed on two sides to the campground's loop road, site 20 feels too open for me. Site 21 is a bit more secluded. It's set at the corner of the campground road with a decent amount of space between it and site 19. It looks like you could drive right through site 22. It's very open to site 20, as well as being on the inside corner of the campground road.

Sites 29, 31, and 32 are all fairly spacious. The wall of woods behind the sites is also filled in with undergrowth, providing a dense barrier against ME 9. The forest on this side of the campground is denser and has thicker undergrowth.

Even though many of the sites here seem exposed to one another, you still won't feel as if you're piled on top of your neighbors. Although you'll certainly be able to see your fellow campers, the sites are generally spacious and situated far enough apart to offer a modicum of elbow room.

You'll have to drive a bit to get to the rest of Bradbury Mountain State Park and the hiking and mountain biking trails, but it's not too far, and it's definitely worth the trip.

KEY INFORMATION

ADDRESS: 528 Hallowell Rd. Pownal, ME 04069

OPERATED BY: Maine Department of Conservation–Bureau of Parks and Lands

INFORMATION: 207-688-4712

OPEN: Year-round

SITES: 35 sites

EACH SITE: Fire ring, picnic table

ASSIGNMENT: First-come, first-served or by reservation: 800-332-1501, 207-624-9950, campwithme.com (additional $2 reservation fee per site, per night)

REGISTRATION: At ranger station as you enter the campground; check in after 1 p.m., check out by 11 a.m.

FACILITIES: Pit toilets, water spigots, recycling station, playground

PARKING: At sites

FEE: Maine residents, $11; nonresidents, $19

RESTRICTIONS: *Pets:* On leash only
Fires: In fire rings
Alcohol: Prohibited
Vehicles: Parking at sites only
Other: No visitors after sunset; quiet hours 10 p.m.–7 a.m.; 14-day maximum stay

MAP

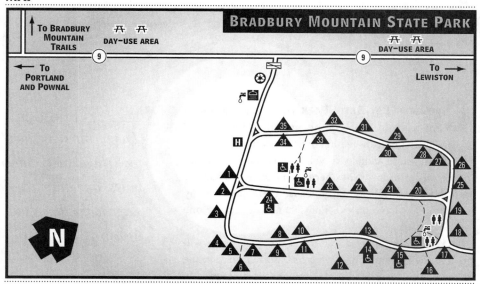

GETTING THERE

Follow ME 9 north through Pownal. Continue heading north, following signs to the campground. You'll pass the other side of Bradbury Mountain State Park before you come to the campground on the right, if you're heading north.

GPS COORDINATES

N43° 54.022036'
W70° 10.688860'

4
COBSCOOK BAY STATE PARK

COBSCOOK BAY STATE PARK comes the closest of any park in this book to providing the remote, oceanside, wilderness feeling of island camping without requiring you to actually travel to an island. You'll find numerous waterfront sites here, all of them spectacular and dramatically beautiful. Because there are so many of them, you have an excellent chance of scoring one of these pristine sites.

When you do get a waterfront site, you'll bear witness to the extreme tidal swing in this area. In fact, the name *Cobscook* is from the Maliseet and Passamaquoddy dialect for "boiling tides." The change in tidal depth runs from 24 to 28 feet! Be extremely careful if you venture out onto the mudflats at low tide to dig up some clams (which is perfectly legal, by the way—up to a peck a day). When the tide turns, it comes *racing* in.

There are several tent-only areas within Cobscook Bay State Park. As you may well imagine, these are the spots you want. The Cobscook Point, Broad Cove, and Harbor Point areas are reserved for our tent-bound brethren. The other areas here are fine, but the tent-only areas are superb.

Cobscook Point includes sites 40 through 74, all carved out of the dense forest of balsam and birch overlooking the waters of Cobscook Bay. These sites are extremely remote, quiet, and scenic, especially the waterfront sites like 40, 41, 44, and 49. Site 43 is set on a small hill with a dramatic view of the bay through the trees, and beautiful breezes blow through the site.

Site 48 requires a short hike in, giving it an amazing sense of seclusion but not much of a view of the bay. That's not a bad tradeoff—depends on what you're in the mood for. Sites 50 and 52 are also set deep within a dense forest of mostly spruce trees for a cool, sylvan feeling.

At the end of Cobscook Point is a short peninsula with sites 56 through 62 (although sites are occasionally taken

> *The picturesque shoreline, waterfront sites, numerous inlets, and dramatic tidal surge make this a unique treasure.*

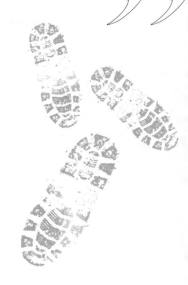

RATINGS

Beauty: ✩ ✩ ✩ ✩ ✩
Privacy: ✩ ✩ ✩ ✩ ✩
Spaciousness: ✩ ✩ ✩ ✩
Quiet: ✩ ✩ ✩ ✩ ✩
Security: ✩ ✩ ✩ ✩
Cleanliness: ✩ ✩ ✩ ✩ ✩

ADDRESS: RR 1, Box 127
Dennysville, ME
04628

OPERATED BY: Maine Department
of Conservation–
Bureau of Parks
and Lands

INFORMATION: 207-726-4412

OPEN: May 15–Oct. 15

SITES: 106 sites

EACH SITE: Fire ring,
picnic table

ASSIGNMENT: First-come, first-
served or by
reservation: 800-
332-1501, 207-624-
9950, campwithme
.com (additional $2
reservation fee per
site, per night)

REGISTRATION: At ranger station
as you enter park

FACILITIES: Flush toilets, water
spigots, pay show-
ers, picnic area,
public boat launch

PARKING: At sites

FEE: Maine residents,
$14; nonresidents,
$24

RESTRICTIONS: *Pets:* On leash only
Fires: In established
fireplaces only
Alcohol: Prohibited
Vehicles: Parking at
sites only
Other: Quiet hours
10 p.m.–7 a.m.;
14-day maximum
stay; check in after
1 p.m., check out
by 11 a.m.; limit
of 1 peck of clams
per day

out of use to allow for regrowth). These are incredibly secluded. This area is reminiscent of the revered (at least by me) Peninsula A at the Mount Desert Campground. Site 56, the first site you'll come to, requires a hike of 50 or so yards. Very large and surrounded by dense woods, this site would be perfect for a larger group or family.

The rest of the sites on the end of Cobscook Point—57, 59, and 62—are at the water's edge. They are moderately spacious and extraordinarily secluded from each other. All these sites share a common parking area as you head out onto the peninsula.

Back on the campground loop road, sites 63, 64, and 65 are also set along the water's edge, and are far enough from each other to offer some seclusion. Sites 66 and 67 are spectacularly secluded hike-in waterside sites, about 50 feet from the road. Site 72 is on a hill off the inside of the road, so it offers a nice sense of seclusion, but you miss the commanding view of the bay afforded by some of the other sites.

Farther along the main campground road heading toward Harbor Point and Whiting Bay, you'll find sites 33, 34, and 35, which are open to the road but next to a small pond that is quite scenic. These sites are also close to the day-use access for the clam flats. You won't find fresher seafood than clams that were deep in the briny mud just a couple of hours ago.

The cozy Harbor Point area is home to sites 29 through 32. Site 29, at the end of a long, grassy drive-way, is a fairly open site with sweeping views of the bay. Site 30 is on a bluff overlooking the bay. Sites 31 and 32 are nicely private and set along the shore of the bay. All the Harbor Point sites are quite secluded from each other, so there really isn't a bad one here. Site 30 is the best, as it is extraordinarily isolated and affords a price-less view of Cobscook Bay.

Broad Cove is another of Cobscook Bay State Park's tent-only areas with a plethora of beautiful hike-in and waterside sites. Sites 75, 77, 78, and 79 are hike-in sites that are spectacularly secluded and give you that feeling of being deep in the woods. Sites 83 and 84 are also nicely isolated hike-in sites that share a parking area. If you can't score a waterfront site, do what you can to land one of these.

Sites 85 and 86 share a parking area as well, but these hike-in sites are set down on the water from site 89, so they are incredibly private and scenic. It's a short walk down toward the water, but the site itself is not as close to the water as sites 85, 86, and 88. Sites 90, 92, 95, and 96 are also spectacular waterside sites with short walks in to them.

Then you come to site 101. This is one of those to-die-for campsites. The hike in is about 200 feet, making it a bit challenging to haul in your gear, but the sense of solitude is worth it. You'll hike up and down rolling terrain and over a short bridge to reach this profoundly secluded site. It's set within some fairly dense forest, but it's on a bluff over-looking the bay, so you'll get slivers of bay view and fantastic sea breezes.

As you head toward the day-use area, most of the sites include covered picnic tables, which would be nice on a rainy day. Sites 102 and 103 are set off on their own and also have covered picnic tables. Site 111 is another nice hike-in site in this area. Sites 114 and 115 are set off on their own. They're fairly close together but very secluded from the other sites. Site 116 stands alone, offering a deep sense of privacy. Site 119 sits at an intersection of the campground road and is open to the road, but there are no other sites around; it also overlooks a wildflower meadow that separates the camping area from the day-use area, so it's quite scenic. Sites 124 and 125 are very secluded, with water views.

The Whiting Bay area, home to sites 1 through 27, is designated as the RV zone, but it still has some nice sites with good tent-camping potential. These sites are fairly large and private, so don't panic if you pick one and hear an RV lumbering toward you.

After you pass site 27, you'll come to the loops for sites 1 through 8 and 9 through 26. Site 2 is a medium-sized site on an open, grassy spot with an amazing view of the bay through loosely spaced spruce trees. Site 3 is very large and perched on a bluff overlooking the bay for gorgeous views and sea breezes.

Most of the sites on the outer edge of the loop have D-shaped driveways to facilitate egress for the land yachts. That also makes them very spacious for tent campers. Site 4 has awesome views, but it's quite open to the road. Site 5 is a pleasant, open spot set down from the road. It's very open to the bay for dramatic views and breezes, but it's also close to the restrooms. Sites 6 through 8 are set in their own little loop. They are slightly open but have fantastic bay views.

A few other sites here are worth exploring. Site 17 is small and open to the road, but it's right next to a trail that leads down to the shore. Site 18 is very spacious and offers a decent sense of privacy because it's secluded from the road and from neighboring sites. Site 22 is large and has that D-shaped driveway, so it's secluded from the road by an "island" of trees and shrubs that form the center of the D.

There's only one thing that bothered me about the Cobscook Bay State Park experi-ence: I can't for the life of me figure out how many clams constitute a peck.

MAP

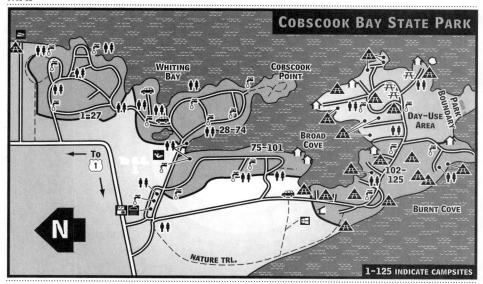

COBSCOOK BAY STATE PARK

WHITING BAY

COBSCOOK POINT

1-27

28-74

75-101

BROAD COVE

DAY-USE AREA

PARK BOUNDARY

To 1

102-125

BURNT COVE

N

NATURE TRL.

1-125 INDICATE CAMPSITES

GETTING THERE

Follow US 1 north for what seems like an eternity. Cobscook Bay State Park is on the right, in the town of Dennysville.

GPS COORDINATES

N44° 50.987399'
W67° 9.471095'

5 HERMIT ISLAND CAMPGROUND

YOU CAN ADD **HERMIT ISLAND** to your list of favorites right away, even if you've never been here. It has some spectacular oceanfront sites. On its campground map, Hermit Island marks sites as Ocean Prime, Prime, Choice, and Value. Generally speaking, you'll be in pretty good shape following those guidelines. They're an honest and accurate assessment of the "wow" factor of the sites, although even the Value sites are nicely wooded and secluded. The Ocean Prime sites are absolutely breathtaking. Do yourself a favor and reserve one well in advance.

This is a fairly large campground, with 275 sites. They're numbered according to the road upon which they're located, sort of like Wompatuck State Park in Massachusetts (see page 198). When you're selecting a site or making a reservation, be sure to specify both the road and the site number.

The Joe's Head Road sites are among the top Ocean Prime spots. Sites 3 and 4 are a bit open but set against windswept dunes and beach undergrowth. Sites 1 and 2 are nicely secluded right on the beach. Try, try, try to get one of these sites. If you do, you'll be glad you did and you'll never want to leave. The sites have a sandy surface and are surrounded by dense beach undergrowth. They're open to the beach as well, so you'll fall asleep to the sound of the crashing surf.

Joe's Head site 10 is nicely secluded right on the beach. You couldn't ask for a more perfect beachfront site. Sites 11 and 12 are higher on a bluff. Sites 8 and 9 are set back from the beach and bluff. They're very spacious yet a bit open to each other. They'd make a great pair of sites for a larger group.

The Ocean Sweep sites are also incredible. As the name implies, these sites sit on a bluff, offering amazing views of the ocean and cool ocean breezes. Site 7 is set back from the edge of the bluff and is more shaded.

> *Hermit Island has it all—beachfront sites and densely wooded sites. And best of all, they're on an island.*

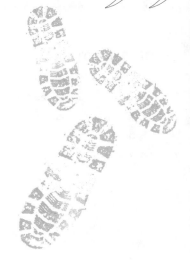

RATINGS

Beauty: ☆ ☆ ☆ ☆ ☆
Privacy: ☆ ☆ ☆ ☆
Spaciousness: ☆ ☆ ☆ ☆
Quiet: ☆ ☆ ☆ ☆
Security: ☆ ☆ ☆ ☆
Cleanliness: ☆ ☆ ☆ ☆

ADDRESS:	6 Hermit Island Rd. Phippsburg, ME 04562 (office: 42 Front St., Bath, ME 04530)
OPERATED BY:	Hermit Island Campground
INFORMATION:	207-443-2101, hermitisland.com
OPEN:	Mid-May–mid-Oct. (full operation late June–Labor Day, limited facilities and reduced rates in off-season)
SITES:	275 sites
EACH SITE:	Loose-rock fireplace, picnic table
ASSIGNMENT:	At check-in at campground headquarters
REGISTRATION:	By reservation (by mail beginning in January and by mail or phone beginning in February) or first-come, first-served (after Labor Day)
FACILITIES:	Flush toilets, showers, composting toilets, boat launch
PARKING:	At campsites
FEE:	$35–$60 per night, depending on site and season
RESTRICTIONS:	*Pets:* Not allowed *Fires:* In fireplaces *Alcohol:* At campsites *Vehicles:* 1 per campsite (no visitors) *Other:* 2 adults and 2 children or 4 adults and no children per site, check in after 2 p.m., check out by 10 a.m.

Sites 5 and 6 are phenomenal and open up to dramatic ocean views.

Dune Way is home to some Prime sites just off the water. They're still very close to the beach, though. These sites are quite spacious and nicely secluded from each other, carved out of dense beach undergrowth.

The West Dune Way sites are a bit more open. Set on a sandy surface, site 57 is huge and secluded. Site 59 is a bit more secluded still, while site 58 is fairly open. Site 60 is huge and fairly private. Sites 61, 62, and 63 sit higher on the bluff, offering beautiful views and ocean breezes. Site 64 is fabulously secluded, with a dramatic view of the ocean.

West Dune Way sites 66, 66W, and 66N are all well off the road. These are some top-notch sites—some of the best at Hermit Island, and that's saying something! Site 66W has to be one of the best in terms of seclusion, view, and proximity to the beach. West Dune Way site 69 is also nicely secluded, set in a fairly dense forest. Site 70 is also wonderfully secluded. It's a long, narrow site that affords a deeper sense of privacy.

On Bayberry, a short crossroad heading off Island Road, sites 14 and 19 are nicely secluded in the dense undergrowth. Site 14 is a bit open to site 22, which is also set on a sandy surface—it's truly like camping on the beach. Overall, the closer to the water you are here at Hermit Island, the better off you'll be.

Sites 20 and 21 on Bayberry are both secluded sites tucked down off the road. Site 23 is set a bit farther back. Sites 24 and 25 are also up on a bluff overlooking the water. Site 27 here has sweeping ocean views. The sites here are set on a bluff overlooking the water. Site 32 is fairly secluded; it's near sites 30 and 31, which would also make a nice pair of sites.

Heading back down Island Road, you'll find site 49, which is quite spacious and secluded, with good water views. Sites 50 through 52 are nice on-the-water sites. Sites 51 and 52 are a good pair of sites for a larger group. Site 50 is spectacular—very scenic and situated on the water. You can set up your tent beneath a canopy of hemlock.

On Western Reach, sites 11 and higher are somewhat smaller, but they're well secluded and set on a bluff, with sweeping views of the bay and ocean breezes. Sites 12 and 13 have panoramic views of water. Sites 15 and 16 are a bit more open to each other but are still incredibly scenic.

The twisty road called Cross Island is home to more Choice sites and also the trailheads for the Blue, Orange, and Red trails. Site 7 is set in an airy grove of birch and nicely secluded. Site 6 is very secluded. It's also situated within a birch grove but has a dense forest behind it. Site 5 is also fairly well secluded, set at a bend in the road. Cross Island sites 1 through 4 are all on a bluff, yielding commanding views and steady ocean breezes—these are also among the finest of Hermit Island's sites.

Back down to the island interior, the Iris Downs sites are wide open to each other. These would make good spots for a huge group or family reunion. On the other hand, site 55, which is just next to this area, is nicely secluded by dense undergrowth. On Dune Way heading back to Island Road, sites 45 and 46 are nicely set off in the dense forest and are very well shaded.

Over on East Tack, site 1 is huge and private. It's right on the water, facing The Branch. It's a bit less breezy and a bit more wooded than the oceanfront sites but beautifully scenic nonetheless. Site 2 is a little more open, but it still has a nice sense of privacy. The rest of the East Tack sites are fairly open, but they're also right on the water.

Harbor Grove Road hosts several smaller sites right on the water. They're also tucked into a dense forest of pine and maple. Site 2 is smallish but set on the water overlooking The Branch. Sites 4 and 5 are off the water but are still nice sites. Site 6 is set on the water within a loose grove of maple and pine.

On the water and a bit farther down from the road, site 7 is more secluded. Site 8 is large and offers a decent sense of seclusion. Site 9, a private water site, tumbles down to the harbor's edge. Sites 12, 13, and 15 are fairly open but in a dramatic waterfront setting.

The Branch water sites are fairly open to each other but right on the water, so that's hard to beat. The inland sites have nice water views with a similar sense of openness. Sites 7 through 9 are under a dense forest canopy, so they feel a bit more secluded. Site 6 is a bit larger, with sweeping water views. Site 5, on the Branch road, is beautiful, open to the sky and the water. The forest is a bit denser over Site 4, so that's a nice shady site. Site 3 is on the waterside but up off the water a bit.

Hermit Island has it all: beachfront sites on the sand amid dense, hardy shrubs; sites overlooking the bay high on a bluff; densely wooded sites encircled by forest—and best of all, they're all on an island. Check this place out and it's sure to become one of your favorites.

MAP

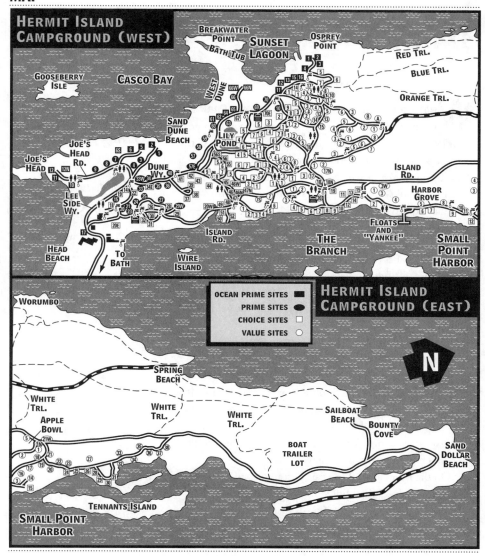

GETTING THERE

Follow US 1 to Bath. (As you head north, do not cross the Bath Bridge.) Then follow ME 209 and ME 216 out to Hermit Island.

GPS COORDINATES

N43° 43.206854'
W69° 51.134055'

6
LAMOINE
STATE PARK

Ellsworth

WHAT DO YOU DO WHEN ACADIA NATIONAL PARK is packed? Head a bit farther north to Lamoine State Park, which is just far enough away to allow you to escape the swarms of Acadia-area campers and travelers during the summer. Most of the sites at the park, which overlooks the waters of Frenchman Bay toward Bar Harbor, have a very open feel.

The view of the ocean and the nearly constant cool breezes give Lamoine State Park an easy combination of pastoral serenity and seaside appeal. The whole gestalt here is that of being on a windswept, coastal bluff—which you are! It's a bit different from the wooded campgrounds to which I usually gravitate, but wild and beautiful nevertheless.

The loop road encircling the campground is intersected by several short roads that run parallel to the seashore. The sites on the outer edge of the loop as you enter the campground, including sites 3, 4, 6, 8, and 9 through 12, are spacious and open, set on a grassy surface and separated by short stands of trees and shrubs. These sites are sunny, breezy, and open, but they don't offer much in the way of privacy.

On the other side of the campground road, the sites are a bit more secluded but still have an open feel. The only trouble here would be if an RV settled in nearby—you would have it right in view. Otherwise, the sites themselves are exposed but comfortable.

Sites 10 through 13 are open but also secluded from each other by short stands of deciduous trees and solid undergrowth. The backs of these sites open to a huge field and the group camping area—a great spot for stargazing on a clear night.

As you move down this side of the campground, there's more of a sense of solitude to sites 13 and 14, set along the outer edge of the campground loop road. Site 14 is encircled by dense deciduous forest. Situated within

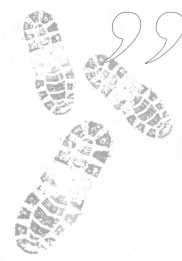

> *During the thick of summer, when Acadia is mobbed, head north to Lamoine State Park to reclaim the solitude for which Maine is renowned.*

RATINGS

Beauty: ✿ ✿ ✿ ✿
Privacy: ✿ ✿ ✿
Spaciousness: ✿ ✿ ✿
Quiet: ✿ ✿ ✿ ✿
Security: ✿ ✿ ✿ ✿ ✿
Cleanliness: ✿ ✿ ✿ ✿

KEY INFORMATION

ADDRESS: 23 State Park Rd. Ellsworth, ME 04605

OPERATED BY: Maine Department of Conservation– Bureau of Parks and Lands

INFORMATION: 207-667-4778

OPEN: Mid-May–Oct. 15

SITES: 62

EACH SITE: Fire ring, picnic table

ASSIGNMENT: First-come, first-served or by reservation: 800-332-1501, 207-624-9950, campwithme .com (additional $2 reservation fee per site, per night)

REGISTRATION: At ranger station as you enter campground

FACILITIES: Hot showers, flush toilets, water spigots

PARKING: At sites

FEE: Maine residents, $15; nonresidents, $25

RESTRICTIONS: *Pets:* On leash only
Fires: In fire rings only
Alcohol: Prohibited
Vehicles: Parking at sites only
Other: Quiet hours 10 p.m.–7 a.m.; 14-day maximum stay; check in after 1 p.m., check out by 11 a.m.

a loose grove of spruce and backed into the mixed forest, site 15 is open with a delightful wooded-grove feel. It's right at a campground-road intersection, but it has a comfortable, charming character.

Heading back toward the campground entrance on one of the intersecting roads brings you to the sites numbered in the high teens and low 20s, which have an exposed feel but are secluded on the sides. Sites 23 through 25 are right at the corner intersection of the campground road.

A number of wide-open field sites lie in the center of the campground at Lamoine State Park, including most of the sites in the 30s. These don't provide much privacy, although some are somewhat isolated on the sides. They're also fairly close to (and within view of) the shower building.

Sites 16 and 17 are tiny but cozy and very secluded. They're carved out of a very dense forest of short deciduous trees and thick undergrowth.

Site 41 is wide open to the road but secluded from its neighbors. You're getting closer to the water here, so you have tantalizing views of the bay through the trees. Site 44, unfortunately, is way too exposed and right behind the restroom building. Site 43 opens to site 42 and the restrooms, but it's secluded on the sides and offers views of the bay to balance the restroom view.

The sites that open to the water are where you really want to be at Lamoine State Park. Sites 56 through 62 are set along the campground road facing the open view of the ocean. The views of Frenchman Bay and its islands are worthy of the Rockefellers. The view from sites 57 through 60 is through loose crabapple and maple trees growing in the picnic area. From 61 and 62, you view the bay through a majestic stand of spruce. There's also a short path down to the water right next to site 62. You can also get to the 1-mile Loop Trail.

All these sites are spacious and open to the road, but they're also open to the view, and they're fairly well secluded from each other. Sites 58 and 59 probably feel the most isolated and farthest from their neighbors. Each is surrounded on three sides by dense undergrowth and shrubs. They open to the bay view through a grove of loosely spaced spruce and pine, trees of hardy stock that stand up to the steady salty breezes.

MAP

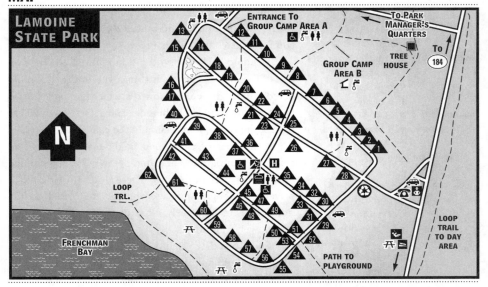

The scent here is that potent Maine blend of ever-green forest and salty ocean tang, topped with a bit of wood smoke as the day draws to an end. Take a moment after you've set up your campsite to sit back, draw in a deep breath, and enjoy the sights, sounds, and smells of this oceanside campground.

GETTING THERE

Follow US 1 north through Ellsworth. At the junction of US 1 and ME 184, follow ME 184 south to the park.

GPS COORDINATES

N44° 27.239206'
W68° 17.889490'

7
LILY BAY
STATE PARK

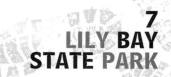

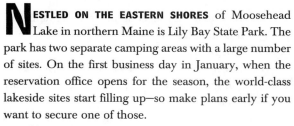

> *Lily Bay State Park is just one facet of the north Maine Woods jewel that is Moosehead Lake.*

NESTLED ON THE EASTERN SHORES of Moosehead Lake in northern Maine is Lily Bay State Park. The park has two separate camping areas with a large number of sites. On the first business day in January, when the reservation office opens for the season, the world-class lakeside sites start filling up—so make plans early if you want to secure one of those.

The Dunn Point Area hosts several secluded sites. Drive up a short road to the right and you'll find site 245 tucked off on its own. Just past the entrance to the site, at the end of its "driveway," is a trailhead for the 1.6-mile hiking trail that leads to Rowell Cove.

The sense of solitude at sites 200 and 201 is priceless. These are moderately spacious and very isolated walk-in tent sites. Getting to them requires a short (20- to 30-foot) hike. Both sites are set on a bluff that overlooks the lake, and the views from here are positively epic.

Farther along this same bluff, site 202 is less exposed to the views and the breeze but still offers sliver views of the lake vista and the hills beyond, through the woods. Site 203 is the last site in this cluster on the bluff. It's very spacious, and the breezes and views filter through a wall of conifers.

A trail leads to the lake's beach just before you get to sites 205 and 206. Site 205 is massive. Across the campground road, site 206 is much smaller but very well secluded in dense forest. Sites 207 and 208 are moderately roomy and private.

At site 210, the forest opens again to the lake. This site is isolated on one side by a two-level wall of young and old white pines, along with some other coniferous trees. The forest opens dramatically at the opposite side of the site, allowing for sweeping views of the lake through the loosely spaced trees that pepper the site down to the water's edge.

RATINGS

Beauty: ☆ ☆ ☆ ☆ ☆
Privacy: ☆ ☆ ☆ ☆ ☆
Spaciousness: ☆ ☆ ☆ ☆
Quiet: ☆ ☆ ☆ ☆ ☆
Security: ☆ ☆ ☆ ☆ ☆
Cleanliness: ☆ ☆ ☆ ☆ ☆

Set within a loose grove of conifers, sites 211 and 212 are relatively spacious and overlook the lake. Sites 213 through 215 require a short walk and are all on the lake. These sites are jewels, with a perfect mix of forest and lakeshore. It's well worth the short haul. Not that you'll be able to take your eyes off the lake for long, but these sites are also fairly isolated from each other.

It's very quiet throughout the campground. All you'll hear is the soft splash of the lake and the cool rush of wind through the trees.

You might want to avoid sites 216 and 220, as they're a bit close to the restrooms. Site 218 is large and mildly secluded, with a view of the lake.

The next group of walk-in tent sites includes sites 221 through 224. These are completely secluded from the rest of the campground and moderately secluded from each other. They share the same clear view of the lake as sites 213 through 215.

So by now you must think you have to be right on the waters of Moosehead Lake to have one of Lily Bay's primo sites, eh? Well, wait until you see site 231. It's incredibly spacious, set on a small knoll in the middle of the forest, and absolutely secluded from neighbors on all sides and from the campground road. Its added elevation will help you catch some of the onshore breezes. Just outside the site, a trail leads down to the beach.

The forest encircling the site is characteristic of the area's fantastically diverse population of mature spruce, birch, and maple. Several smaller white pine trees stand to the left as you enter the site. Encircled by forest, this spot feels deeper in the Maine wilderness than you might expect.

A shared entryway brings you to sites 235 and 236. This would make a good pair of sites for a larger group or family needing two sites—if you can't score two magical lakeside sites. Another option for families is site 240, which has a U-shaped driveway you could pull right through. Those two openings do leave it fairly exposed to the road, though.

The Rowell Cove Area also has some dramatic lakeside walk-in tent sites. Sites 33 through 38 are hike-in tent sites perched along a craggy peninsula that recalls the

KEY INFORMATION

ADDRESS: HC 76, Box 425 Greenville, ME 04441

OPERATED BY: Maine Department of Conservation– Bureau of Parks and Lands

INFORMATION: 207-695-2700 or 207-941-4014

OPEN: May 15–Oct. 15

SITES: 86

EACH SITE: Stone hearth or fire ring, picnic table

ASSIGNMENT: First-come, first-served or by reservation: 800-332-1501, 207-624-9950, campwithme .com (additional $2 reservation fee per site, per night)

REGISTRATION: At ranger station as you enter campground

FACILITIES: Pit toilets, water spigots, boat launch, swim area, playground

PARKING: At sites

FEE: Maine residents, $14; nonresidents, $24

RESTRICTIONS: *Pets:* On leash only
Fires: In fire rings only
Alcohol: Prohibited
Vehicles: Parking at sites only
Other: Quiet hours 10 p.m.–7 a.m.; 14-day maximum stay; check in after 1 p.m., check out by 11 a.m.

MAP

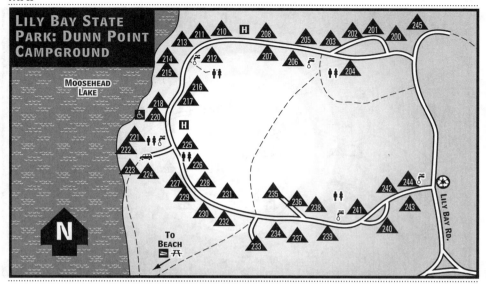

LILY BAY STATE PARK: DUNN POINT CAMPGROUND

MOOSEHEAD LAKE

N

To BEACH

LILY BAY RD.

revered Peninsula A at the eponymous campground on Mount Desert Island. Site 33 is the largest of the group.

You'll enjoy ample views of the lake through loose trees from sites 20 and 21. They're also nicely secluded by dense spruce just open enough to view the lake. Sites 25 and 28 each have a nice sense of solitude, plus a slice of the lake view through the forest.

Several massive conifers frame one side of site 26. The inside loop sites in this part of the campground are fairly well secluded from each other, while sites 29 and 30 are both open to the campground loop road. These two sites are also near the parking for sites 39 through 41.

The cluster of sites that includes 39 through 46 is another majestic spot. These sites are all spacious, set right on the lake within a small cove and beneath a loosely spaced grove of spruce trees. The floor is a soft bed of pine needles over a firm, sandy surface. The sites are open to the lake, with exceptional breezes and views. The walking distance to the sites ranges from 50 to 70 feet.

Site 31 opens right to the parking area and feels too exposed. Site 32 is huge and very secluded. It's surrounded by a thick wall of forest and further isolated because it's a bit farther down the campground road.

The lower-numbered sites here aren't quite as impressive, but they aren't bad. Even though it's set right where the campground loop road rejoins itself, site 8 is spacious and isolated. Site 7 is similar, with glimpses of the lake. Site 5 feels very exposed, being open to the road, but it has a fabulous view of the lake.

MAP

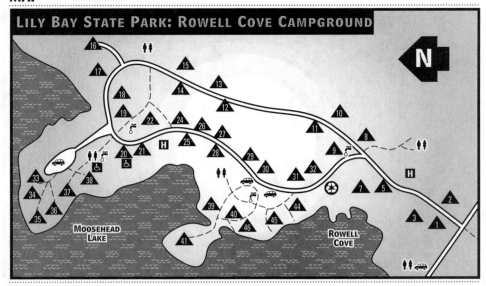

LILY BAY STATE PARK: ROWELL COVE CAMPGROUND

N

MOOSEHEAD LAKE

ROWELL COVE

Follow ME 6 north to Greenville. From Greenville, take Lily Bay Road off to the right and follow it to the park.

It may be tiny and exposed to the road, but site 12 is set way off from any neighboring sites. Site 13 has a similar character. It's carved out of fairly dense forest. Site 14 is spacious, secluded, punctuated by three massive spruce trees, and encircled by dense, mixed forest.

You have glimpses and slivers of lake view through the forest here near the sites in the upper teens. Site 15 is open to the road and close to the restrooms. Site 16 is colossal and tucked well off the campground loop road for a deep sense of solitude. Site 17 is large and set off from its neighbors, but it's a bit open to the road. It's also very open to the sky, and the lake is visible from the site.

GPS COORDINATES

ROWELL COVE
N45° 34.619493'
W69° 32.997544'

DUNN POINT
N45° 34.351351'
W69° 33.629079'

8
MOUNT BLUE STATE PARK

> *There's a dense, diverse forest covering the campground at Mount Blue State Park, whose lush quality recalls a rainforest.*

MOUNT BLUE STATE PARK is actually a pair of parks. One section lies on Mount Blue itself, while the other section is down alongside Webb Lake. The trails on and around the 3,187-foot Mount Blue and Tumbledown, Little Jackson, Blueberry, and Bald mountains are suitable for hikers of all abilities. There's also a multiuse trail in the Center Hill section of the park for mountain bikers, hikers, equestrians, and ATVs.

The park's campground is in the Webb Lake section. All 134 sites lie within a fairly short walk of the lake and are set within a dense, diverse forest with thick undergrowth. The woods are a mix of young and old deciduous and coniferous trees, with lots of spruce, birch, and maple.

While the forest varies dramatically, the sites here have a relatively standard shape and layout, though they differ in size. Surprisingly, it's not the quietest place in the world. As I set up camp at Mount Blue, the density of the forest provided a pleasant sense of seclusion, but I found that sound traveled through the forest quite freely. After dinner, when night settles in, the campground quiets right down, but during the day you'll hear noise from surrounding campsites.

As you enter the camping area, sites 1 through 10 are spread along the main campground road. The remaining sites are grouped in two loops. The first 10 sites are quite spacious but very open to the road. A fair amount of traffic drives by—as everyone going in and out of the campground has to pass these sites. Within this cluster of sites, Site 1 is actually the most secluded, thanks to the forest at the site's edge. It's still quite close to the road, however. Sites 4 and 5 have a pretty solid barrier of trees buffering them from the road, but sites 7 and 8 are exposed.

The forest enshrouding the loop with sites 11 through 78 is populated primarily by moderately tall spruce and deciduous trees. The trees aren't huge, but they are

RATINGS

Beauty: ✩ ✩ ✩ ✩
Privacy: ✩ ✩ ✩ ✩
Spaciousness: ✩ ✩ ✩ ✩
Quiet: ✩ ✩ ✩
Security: ✩ ✩ ✩ ✩
Cleanliness: ✩ ✩ ✩ ✩

numerous and crowded with undergrowth. There is an almost primeval feel to the forest that translates into a wonderful sense of seclusion at most of these sites. The sites are very clean and well kept. Some have a bit more forest buffering them from their neighbors, especially sites 15 and 17. Site 19 and the sites in the lower 20s are more tightly packed than those in the rest of this loop, but encircled by thick woods.

A trail leads down to the lake between sites 26 and 28. Set a good distance from site 30 at a bend in the road, site 31 is tucked into a dense stand of trees, so it offers an additional measure of privacy.

Site 34 is small, but it feels isolated within a bucolic grove where spruces tower above a thick blanket of ferns. Surrounded by dense deciduous forest with plenty of room between it and the next site, site 35 maintains a marvelously secluded feel.

Sites 38, 40, and 41 are set within a mature forest of tall maples and birch. The loose arrangement of trees in this part of the campground lets more sunlight filter down. Site 44 is colossal. You could land a space shuttle here, if that's how you happened to arrive at the campground.

Though they vary in size, sites 47 through 77 share a similar layout. They are also uniformly spaced. Site 54, in a loose grove of tall spruce, is large and open to the sky. A trail heads off to the beach between sites 57 and 58.

Set along the outside of the loop, sites 58 through 62 are spacious and open. Sites 69 and 71 are particularly secluded, distant from their neighbors, and carved out of a dense, deciduous forest with thick undergrowth. Site 69 is only moderately sized, but 71 is huge.

Within the loop containing sites 79 through 136, the forest is crowded with trees and underbrush. The sites are uniformly distributed along the inside and outside of the loop. The space between most sites is roughly equal to that of an average site, affording quite a sense of privacy. Sites 128 and up seem to have slightly more forest between them. There are no hookups in the park, but even if an RV should happen to dock near you, the thick forest in this loop will obscure your view.

A trail to the lake leaves this section between sites 109 and 110. Trails also lead to the centrally located

KEY INFORMATION

ADDRESS: 299 Center Hill Rd. Weld, ME 04285

OPERATED BY: Maine Department of Conservation– Bureau of Parks and Lands

INFORMATION: 207-585-2347 or 207-585-2261

OPEN: May 15–Columbus Day

SITES: 134

EACH SITE: Stone hearth, picnic table

ASSIGNMENT: First-come, first-served or by reservation: 800-332-1501, 207-624-9950, camp withme.com (extra $2 reservation fee per site, per night)

REGISTRATION: At ranger station

FACILITIES: Hot showers, flush toilets, pit toilets, water spigots, boat launch, amphi-theater, sand beach, nature cen-ter, canoe rental, cross-country and snowmobile trails, ice rink

PARKING: At sites

FEE: Maine residents, $15; nonresidents, $25

RESTRICTIONS: *Pets:* On leash only
Fires: In fire rings
Alcohol: Prohibited
Vehicles: Parking at sites only
Other: Quiet hours 10 p.m.–7 a.m.; 14-day maximum stay; check in 1 p.m., check out 11 a.m.

MAP

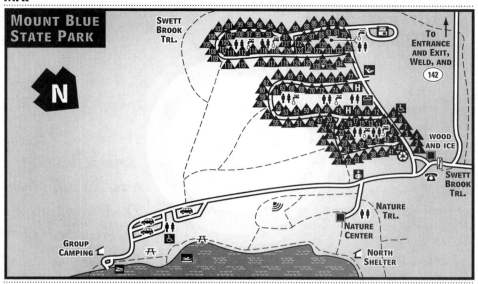

GETTING THERE

From the town of Weld, follow ME 142 to Weld Corner. Follow the signs for the Webb Lake section of Mount Blue State Park.

GPS COORDINATES

N44° 40.924473'
W70° 26.983094'

restrooms spread throughout both site loops. You'll never have to walk very far to find one.

The dense forest at Mount Blue Campground leaves few sites open to the sky. There are a few exceptions to this, sites 44, 54, 93, and 106 among them. If you like to gaze at the night sky, check out one of these sites. Otherwise, once dusk settles, you'll feel enveloped by the deep woods.

9
MOUNT DESERT CAMPGROUND

NESTLED NEAR THE APEX of Somes Sound on Mount Desert Island, Mount Desert Campground provides a tent-camping experience that's as close to perfect as any campground in this book offers. The entire campground is artfully carved out of the rolling woods that reach all the way down to the shoreline. The campground is also conveniently situated near the main entrance to Acadia National Park and right near the Eagle Lake and Witch Hole Pond loops.

Mount Desert doesn't have any areas set aside specifically for tent camping, but there really isn't a bad site in the place. The A-, B-, and C-area sites are the best, especially the contiguous sites on the A peninsula, A12 through A14+ (which accounts for four sites since site A14+ was added). To get to these, you have to walk about 50 feet along the peninsula. If those sites are taken, as is often the case, another piece of prime camping real estate is site A5, on a small bluff overlooking the water.

You're in Maine. You're on an island. Do what you can to get a water site. It's well worth the effort and expense. If you set up somewhere for a night or two and then a water site opens up, it will be worth the trouble to move. Just make sure the site is truly vacant, not reserved, and let the owners know you'd like to relocate.

The waterside sites at Mount Desert follow the undulating terrain as it dives into the headwaters of Somes Sound: beautiful, dramatic, and anything but flat. If you saw the terrain from a distance, you'd wonder how you could ever pitch a tent here.

When you check in at the main entrance, they'll ask you if you need some nails. *Excuse me,* you'll think, *did I somehow volunteer for campground maintenance?* Say yes, though—you'll need them. Every site at the water's edge or on any uneven terrain has a solid wooden deck on which you can set up your tent, using nails in lieu of stakes. If the campground owners hadn't built these tent

> *Perched on the rugged shores at the top of Somes Sound, Mount Desert Campground is nestled in an absolutely pristine setting.*

RATINGS

Beauty: ✪ ✪ ✪ ✪ ✪
Privacy: ✪ ✪ ✪ ✪
Spaciousness: ✪ ✪ ✪ ✪
Quiet: ✪ ✪ ✪ ✪ ✪
Security: ✪ ✪ ✪ ✪ ✪
Cleanliness: ✪ ✪ ✪ ✪ ✪

KEY INFORMATION

ADDRESS: 516 Sound Dr. Mount Desert, ME 04660

OPERATED BY: Owen and Barbara Craighead

INFORMATION: 207-244-3710, mountdesert campground.com

OPEN: Mid-June–Columbus Day (depending on weather); D sites and some E sites close earlier (usually mid-Sept.)

SITES: 161

EACH SITE: Fire pit with grate; most have wooden tent platforms

ASSIGNMENT: Reservations accepted for stays of 1 week or longer, otherwise first-come, first-served

REGISTRATION: At camp headquarters at main entrance

FACILITIES: Restrooms, hot showers, pay phone, camp store, canoe and kayak rentals

PARKING: At or near individual sites

FEE: $29–$52, depending on site and season

RESTRICTIONS: *Pets:* On leash only, before July 1 and after Labor Day
Fires: In fire pits only
Alcohol: At sites only
Vehicles: 1 per site
Other: Check in after 1 p.m., check out by 11 a.m.; maximum 2 adults per site

platforms, they would be lucky to have one or two sites flat enough on which to pitch a tent.

Each area has its own facilities building, with sparkling-clean, well-kept restrooms and coin-operated showers. Here's another hint: even in the summer, the mornings will be cool. Bring more quarters than you think you'll need. Letting the water run stone-cold over a headful of shampoo may cause itchiness, headaches, and loud cursing.

A charming little store on the road leading into the campground sells bundles of firewood; such camping-appropriate groceries as cans of soup and Jiffy Pop popcorn; all sorts of items you may have forgotten, such as batteries and toothpaste; and guidebooks to the hiking trails and carriage roads that take you to some of the island's magical spots. It's also a handy place to pick up a quick cup of coffee and a muffin before you get your own breakfast fire going. You can get some fresh-baked goodies for dessert later that night or make a special trip down with the kids (of any age) for an afternoon ice cream.

Just outside the campground, there's so much to do on Mount Desert Island and in Acadia National Park that you could write an entire book about it. (In fact, people have!) You can hike, bike, paddle, or just find a spot to relax and enjoy the view, which alone can restore your soul. This is classic Maine wilderness, with gentle, rolling, forested mountains sloping right down to the craggy coast. The Atlantic obliges to complete the view with an endless supply of crashing surf.

Rent a canoe or kayak and launch out into Somes Sound, the only fjord on the East Coast. Between the rolling mountains, the rocky shoreline, and the water that glistens like a carpet of diamonds, the paddling is perfect. Just off the dock and boat launch at the campground, you'll paddle past a small island as you enter the sound. This is actually part of Acadia National Park, and atop the tallest pine, in the center of the island, is a bald eagle's nest. On one brilliant August afternoon while paddling out into Somes Sound, I was visited by several pods of brown Atlantic dolphins swimming up the sound. I first heard the quick puff of their breath as they surfaced. It didn't take long to determine the source of the noise once I saw the slender, dark shapes rising

MAP

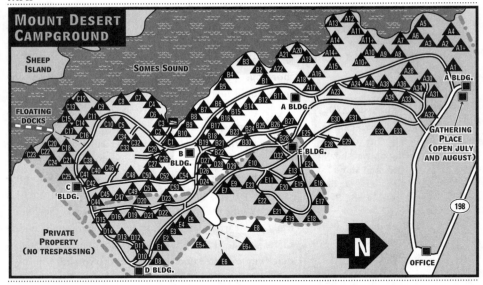

MOUNT DESERT CAMPGROUND

SHEEP ISLAND

SOMES SOUND

FLOATING DOCKS

PRIVATE PROPERTY (NO TRESPASSING)

A BLDG.

B BLDG.

C BLDG.

D BLDG.

E BLDG.

GATHERING PLACE (OPEN JULY AND AUGUST)

198

OFFICE

N

and disappearing into the water in front of me. One of the dolphins actually dove under my kayak and surfaced behind me. I almost tipped over trying to snap a picture of that bold little guy.

Both inside and outside Mount Desert Campground, you can do as much or as little as you like, but you couldn't ask for a more peaceful setting in which to pitch your tent. One cool foggy evening, while kicking back by the campfire, I heard someone playing the flute. The song was Paul Simon's "Duncan." If you're familiar with that tune, you know it has a hauntingly beautiful flute melody. Hearing that echoing throughout the trees, smelling the wood fire, and watching its glowing embers through increasingly sleepy eyes is a memory I will always cherish.

GETTING THERE

From Ellsworth, follow ME 3 onto Mount Desert Island. Follow ME 3 to ME 102/198 south. Stay on ME 198 when it turns left. The campground will be on the right, about a mile after ME 198 splits from ME 102.

GPS COORDINATES

N44° 21.997118'
W68° 19.078889'

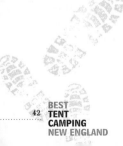

> *The awe-inspiring column of conifers you'll see as you drive into Peaks-Kenny State will put you in the perfect frame of mind for your camping trip.*

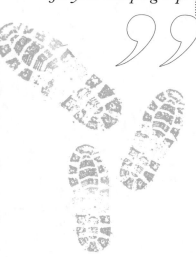

DRIVING INTO PEAKS-KENNY STATE PARK will remind you why we seek out natural places. The long, winding road to the park travels through a corridor of tall, statuesque pines. Following this entryway inspires a feeling of reverence. I found myself involuntarily driving much slower and gazing in awe at the magnificent forest through which this road was carved, and wishing I was already out of my car and walking through the woods.

Peaks-Kenny is an exceptionally quiet and remote campground. All you'll hear is the wind rushing through the treetops. The forest is a dense blend of coniferous and deciduous trees, including numerous birches, lots of dense undergrowth, and large boulders. This area must have been one of the last stops for a southbound glacier a few million years ago.

The sites here have hard, sandy surfaces that hang onto those tent stakes. They're also impeccably clean. The diverse character of the dense forest and the gently rolling topography, peppered with glacial boulders, makes these woodland campsites very scenic and attractive. The 54 sites sit near the shores of Sebec Lake. Most are nicely secluded from the rest, especially on the outer side of the loops. The other sites are a curious blend of solitude and openness.

Site 1 is reminiscent of the drive-in. It resembles a natural cathedral or amphitheater. Its location at the start of the campground loop is unfortunate, however, because it is consequently exposed to the road. Two massive white pines frame the site, and a large boulder declares its rear border. Location aside, this site is spectacular.

Site 6 has a nice open feel and no neighbors, but like site 1, it's quite open to the road. Site 7 feels particularly secluded. It's a huge site set in open woods. Though site 7 is close to one of the campground host

RATINGS

Beauty: ✩✩✩✩✩
Privacy: ✩✩✩✩✩
Spaciousness: ✩✩✩✩
Quiet: ✩✩✩✩✩
Security: ✩✩✩✩
Cleanliness: ✩✩✩✩✩

sites (formerly site 9), the dense forest mutes the sounds of your neighbors.

A long entryway leads into site 8, which is set farther off the campground road. The only drawback to this site is that it's close to the restroom. Site 11 is a bit too open and close to the restrooms as well. Site 10, however, is quite spacious and encircled by a brilliant green wall of deciduous forest.

Site 12 is small but secluded. It's also pitched at a bit of angle, so don't use one of those slippery sleeping pads here or you'll end up in a heap at the bottom of your tent by morning. Likewise, there may not be much space in site 14, but it's way off on its own. The surrounding forest is open, but its location gives it a great sense of solitude.

A boulder garden at the back of site 13 provides solid delineation of the site and adds privacy. It's also fun to climb on, for kids of any age. Sites 15 and 16 are right across the campground road from each other, but they're set apart from the sites on either side. These might be a good choice for a family requiring two sites.

Site 17 is too open to the road, plus it's fairly small. A trail leads to the lake right across from site 19, which is rather exposed and quite close to the bathroom. Site 20 is spacious but feels very open to the road. Site 21 is very well secluded but backs up against the restroom.

Site 23 is very open and up off the road. It's also quite open to the sky for stargazing. The rest of the sites in the 20s are moderately secluded but also convenient to the trail, the lake, and the bathrooms. The sites on the outside of the loop provide the greatest solitude, particularly site 29, which is on the smaller side but is encircled by dense forest and undergrowth.

A tall birch marks the entrance to site 30, and a moderately dense forest of hemlock and mixed deciduous trees surrounds the site. Perched atop a small hill on the campground road, it feels nicely isolated.

Massive hemlock trees frame site 33. It's good-sized but otherwise feels a bit open, and it's right at the intersection of the campground loop road. Site 32 is close to the bathrooms. Site 37 is exposed to the road but otherwise very well secluded, as it's on a small rise and encircled by dense coniferous forest that gives the site a cool, dark, sylvan atmosphere.

KEY INFORMATION

ADDRESS:	Route 1, Box 10 Dover-Foxcroft, ME 04426
OPERATED BY:	Maine Department of Conservation–Bureau of Parks and Lands
INFORMATION:	207-564-2003
OPEN:	Mid-May–Oct. 1
SITES:	54
EACH SITE:	Fire ring, picnic table
ASSIGNMENT:	First-come, first-served or by reservation: 800-332-1501, 207-624-9950, campwithme .com (additional $2 fee per night for reservations)
REGISTRATION:	At ranger station as you enter campground
FACILITIES:	Hot showers, flush toilets, water spigots, canoe rentals
PARKING:	At sites
FEE:	Maine residents, $15; nonresidents, $25
RESTRICTIONS:	*Pets:* On leash only *Fires:* In fire rings *Alcohol:* Not allowed *Vehicles:* At sites *Other:* Quiet hours 10 p.m.–7 a.m., 14-day maximum stay, 2-day minimum for reservations; check in after 1 p.m., check out by 11 a.m.

There is a fantastic sense of seclusion to site 38, which is set back from the campground road amid a dense grove of mostly hemlocks, with a few deciduous trees mixed in. You can barely see this site from the campground road, and vice versa. Site 39 is more open but way down off the road, in its own grove of conifers. Several birch trees frame site 40, which is open to both the campground and the sky.

A curiously arranged wall of boulders backs site 41. One of those boulders has a white pine growing right on top of it. Site 43 has a boulder ledge behind it and sits in a stately stand of hemlocks. Site 46 is way too open for me. It's well off the road but still lacks privacy. Site 47 is kind of small but very well isolated from its neighbors within a moderately dense grove of smaller mixed deciduous and coniferous trees. Sites 48 through 51, especially 49 and 51, are too exposed to the rest of the campground.

Being set off the road gives site 52 a nice sense of privacy and seclusion. A long entryway leads into the site, with just enough of an opening to the sky to allow shafts of sunlight to filter down to this spot. A trail leading to the lake is next to the site entrance.

Site 53 is close to the restrooms. Site 55 is large and well secluded, encircled by a moderately dense, mostly deciduous forest. There's not much undergrowth in this part of the campground, so the forest floor has an open feel.

Several massive boulders block site 56 from view of the road. The site itself is set down off the road as well and is framed on one side by a stand of hemlock and beech trees that further blocks views of the road. The forest opens toward the back of the site, giving it a combined sense of solitude and openness.

Most of the activities in which you'll participate while camping here will be on Sebec Lake—the showcase of Peaks-Kenny State Park. Bring your canoe, kayak, and fishing gear, and you won't have any reason to leave the lake or the campground. Several hiking trails run through the campground as well, including Brown's Point Trail and the Birch Mountain Ledge Trail. Neither of these trails is particularly steep or challenging, so they make for a nice, relaxing hike.

MAP

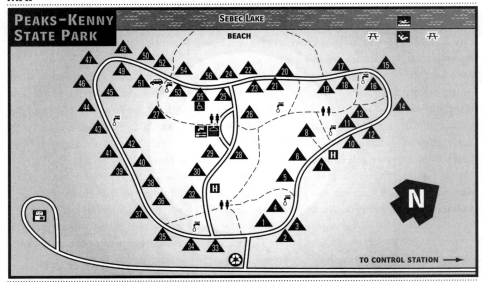

GETTING THERE

Follow ME 153 north from Dover-Foxcroft for about 6 miles until you see signs for the park.

GPS COORDINATES

N45° 15.508468'
W69° 16.651254'

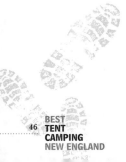

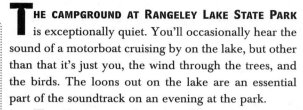

> *Rangeley Lake is the perfect spot if you just want to unplug for a while in the sylvan solitude of northwestern Maine.*

THE CAMPGROUND AT RANGELEY LAKE STATE PARK is exceptionally quiet. You'll occasionally hear the sound of a motorboat cruising by on the lake, but other than that it's just you, the wind through the trees, and the birds. The loons out on the lake are an essential part of the soundtrack on an evening at the park.

The 50 campsites here are spread out around a single large loop. Sites 2, 3, 6, 10, 17, 21, 27, 33, and 42 are first-come, first-served; the rest can be reserved. The sites here are set beneath a dense, truly mixed forest of young and old, deciduous and coniferous trees. A nice amount of forest and space between sites provides a solid sense of seclusion in almost all of them. This is a very remote campground with relatively few sites, so there is lots of privacy and silence.

Site 9 offers a delightfully secluded atmosphere. It's surrounded by a dense forest of birch and spruce trees. Just past site 9, a footpath leads down to the beach on Rangeley Lake. Just past the footpath is a small open field with a playground area and volleyball net. The playground itself is quite scenic, overlooking the lake through the trees.

Site 11 is also extraordinarily secluded. This moderately spacious site is carved out of a dense grove of conifers. All the sites numbered in the teens are actually very well screened from each other. Site 13 is a bit more open, but you can catch brief glimpses of the lake through the woods. Site 17 is very secluded, likewise carved out of the coniferous forest.

A thick wall of forest encircles site 19, but privacy isn't the best aspect of this site. A 50-foot path leads from the site to your own little slice of the lake. This artfully composed lakeside cove has several birch trees growing out over the lake and a short rock jetty leading out from shore. (I suspect some of the other sites on the lake side of the loop also have these little escape routes to the

RATINGS

Beauty: ✩ ✩ ✩ ✩
Privacy: ✩ ✩ ✩ ✩
Spaciousness: ✩ ✩ ✩ ✩
Quiet: ✩ ✩ ✩ ✩ ✩
Security: ✩ ✩ ✩ ✩
Cleanliness: ✩ ✩ ✩ ✩ ✩

water, but I couldn't intrude on my neighbors' sites to find out.)

Another path leads to the lake from site 23. There's a more airy feel here because it's open to the sky and set within a loose grove of young trees. As you come to site 25, the campground road starts to head slightly uphill. Site 26 has a very open, sunny feel and is encircled by a grove of mostly young deciduous trees that form a solid green wall. Site 30 is similarly bright and green. Sites 27 and 29 are quite close to the restrooms, so I'd stay away from these.

Sites 30 and up seem to have a bit more forest between them generally. Though site 33 is small, it's tucked into dense forest and relatively distant from its neighbors—even site 34, which is across the road. Site 34 is back at an angle and screened by a dense stand of trees. This site has a dark, cool feel.

Site 35 affords a solid sense of seclusion, but it's also open to the sky, allowing sunlight to make its way to the site floor. Site 36, like site 34, is nestled in the trees. A large hemlock tree grows to the right of the site as you enter. Site 38 is secluded but very spacious and open to the sky.

The sites on the outside of the loop, including sites 40 and up, have plenty of forest between them for privacy. Most of these sites are also open to the sky, so stargazers take note. Site 42 has a long entryway, which adds to its considerable sense of seclusion.

Site 44 is open to the road and thus has less privacy than most of the other sites at Rangeley Lake. Site 47 is across from the restroom but set back and up from the road in thick mixed forest. Sites 49 and 50 are spacious, but they're situated right where the campground road splits off, and consequently they receive more traffic noise.

Rangeley Lake is pristine. Its remote location in northwestern Maine means it gets a lot less traffic than Sebago Lake farther south in Maine, or Lake Winnipesaukee in New Hampshire. The lake is perfect for whatever draws you to water: canoeing, kayaking, swimming, or fishing. If you're fond of angling, you'll appreciate that Rangeley is renowned for its population of land-locked trout and salmon.

KEY INFORMATION

ADDRESS:	HC 32, Box 5000 Rangeley, ME 04970-5000
OPERATED BY:	Maine Department of Conservation– Bureau of Parks and Lands
INFORMATION:	207-864-3858
OPEN:	Mid-May–Oct. 1
SITES:	50
EACH SITE:	Fire ring, picnic table
ASSIGNMENT:	First-come, first-served or by reservation: 800-332-1501, 207-624-9950, campwithme .com (additional $2 fee per site per night for reservations)
REGISTRATION:	At ranger station as you enter campground
FACILITIES:	Hot showers, flush toilets, playground, boat launch
PARKING:	At sites
FEE:	Maine residents, $15; nonresidents, $25
RESTRICTIONS:	*Pets:* On leash only *Fires:* In established fire rings only *Alcohol:* Not allowed *Vehicles:* Parking at sites only *Other:* Quiet hours 10 p.m.–7 a.m.; 14-day maximum stay; check in after 1 p.m., check out by 11 a.m.

MAP

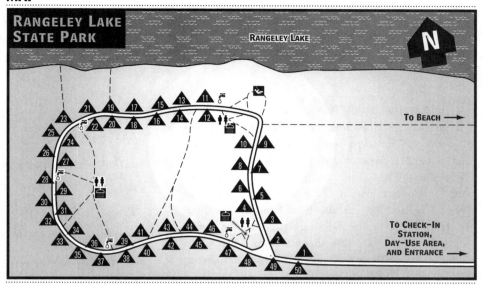

GETTING THERE

Follow ME 4 north from Farmington to Rangeley, and follow the signs to the state park.

GPS COORDINATES

N44° 55.946903'
W70° 42.605381'

There's plenty to do on land here as well. Hiking trails for all abilities abound. Try the nearby 3-mile trail up Bald Mountain, a 2,443-foot peak with commanding views of the lake and the surrounding forests and hills. Within the park, the Moose Country Corridor Trail is a good choice for a short hike with the little ones. As always, the birding and wildlife-viewing in this remote, densely forested part of Maine are unparalleled. When passing any wet, marshy spots in your travels, keep an eye out for moose.

THE **NATIONAL PARK SERVICE MANAGES** two camp-grounds within Acadia National Park: Seawall and Blackwoods. The latter (see page 16) is more popular, and more often crowded, by virtue of its location along the oceanside Park Loop Road. In fact, I've often camped there just for that reason. It's extremely convenient to Park Loop Road's prime attractions, Sand Beach, Thunder Hole (a hole in the rocks carved out by the surf in which the waves cause a thunderous boom), Otter Cliffs, and some great hiking trails up and over the short, steep cliff known as The Beehive.

So I was pleasantly surprised, if not completely converted, the first time I pulled into Seawall Campground. There are three areas to check out here: the drive-in tent sites in areas A and B, and the walk-in tent sites in area D. No tents are allowed in area C, but that's the RV section, so why would I want to be there anyway?

The A loop is set beneath a dense coniferous forest. The character of the forest and the fact that most sites are set well off the road ensure a complete sense of solitude. The campground road runs along two sides and rejoins itself after making a large loop right at site 1, which is a bit open but quite spacious. Site 2 is also spacious, set farther off the road in a dense grove of mixed conifers. Site 3 is tucked into a grove of slender young conifers and is open to the sky. Site 6 is way back from the road and offers isolation. Sites 7 and 8 share an entryway. Site 8 is completely separated from the road, and site 7 is partially private. Site 10 is buffered on the sides, but it's a bit close to the road.

Dense undergrowth surrounds sites 11 and 13, giving them a deep-woods aura. Sites 14 and 15 are airy and abut a clearing. They are open to each other, which may appeal to groups and large families, but fairly secluded from the campground road. Site 16 is set far back in this clearing, farther from the road but open to the field

> *The "village" of walk-in tent sites is reason enough to come camping at Seawall. Its setting on Mount Desert Island and near all of Acadia National Park makes it just that much better.*

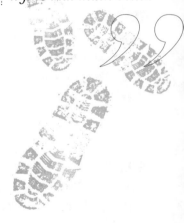

RATINGS

Beauty: ☆ ☆ ☆ ☆
Privacy: ☆ ☆ ☆ ☆
Spaciousness: ☆ ☆ ☆ ☆
Quiet: ☆ ☆ ☆ ☆
Security: ☆ ☆ ☆ ☆
Cleanliness: ☆ ☆ ☆ ☆ ☆

KEY INFORMATION

ADDRESS: 668 Seawall Rd. Southwest Harbor, ME 04679

OPERATED BY: National Park Service

INFORMATION: Acadia National Park, P.O. Box 177, Bar Harbor, ME, 04609; 207-288-3338 or 207-244-3600

OPEN: Late May–Sept. 30

SITES: 205 sites (plus 5 group sites)

EACH SITE: Fire ring, picnic table

ASSIGNMENT: First-come, first-served or by reservation, 877-444-6777 or recreation.gov

REGISTRATION: At ranger station as you enter the campground

FACILITIES: Flush toilets, water spigots

PARKING: At sites and central area within D loop

FEE: $14–$20 (depending on site location); park entrance pass required ($20 weekly, $40 annually)

RESTRICTIONS: *Pets:* On leash only
Fires: In established fire rings only
Alcohol: At sites only
Vehicles: Parking at sites only, or parking areas near D sites
Other: Quiet hours 10 p.m.–7 a.m.; maximum 6 people per site

shared by 14 and 15. A wall of foliage surrounds the field, clearly defining its borders.

Perched at a campground-road intersection as it is, site 20 feels too open to the road. Sites 19 and 22 are set within the woods and way off the road for absolute solitude. Sites 23 through 25 also have moderately long entryways. They are screened by greenery but open to the sky. A long entryway leads to site 31, which is very well secluded but a bit close to the restrooms. Site 33 also has a fairly long "driveway."

Even the sites that feel open here are thoughtfully spaced within the ample, thick forest. The ingenuity of the layout joins the beauty of the setting to complete your experience of sylvan solitude. Another positive element of this campground's design is that site 27 is intended for wheelchair access.

Site 35 is a prime example of the smart layout at Seawall, placed so it's unseen from the road. This site is fantastically secluded and set within dense hemlocks. Sites 36 and 38, however, are a bit open to the road.

A more loosely spaced forest predominates along the B loop, at least at the forest-floor level. There's much less undergrowth, and the forest is populated with older spruce and hemlock that are bare halfway up the trunks, so you have an airy feeling on the ground with a soothing, evergreen canopy overhead. The mostly coniferous forest here imparts a heady perfume—a lingering spicy, tangy scent.

Site 3 is tucked into the trees off the road. Site 5 is a bit small and open, and sites 6 and 7 are very exposed to the road. Sites 8 through 11 are moderately secluded from each other. These sites are all quite spacious and set within a stately hemlock grove.

Sites 12 and 13 are very open to each other and somewhat open to the road. However, these sites are huge, so they're perfect for a group needing two contiguous sites. Sites 15 and 16 are another good pair, although they're a bit smaller. The large sites 21 and 22 share an entryway and are fairly open to each other.

Site 19 enjoys solitude, being well off the road. Site 26 is very spacious and fairly distant from the campground road. Note, however, that sites 23 and 24 are very open to the road and the Dumpster, of all things. I don't know of anyone who would want a dump lurking just outside their campsite. Also, site 27 is oddly positioned just outside the B loop and sees passing traffic.

Generally, the spaciousness of the forest in the B loop doesn't mean a lack of privacy, though you will see your neighbors. It's more like you're nestled within the deep woods. There's a comforting openness to the forest floor, the moss-and-fern ground cover lending a rainforest feel to the woods. The dense, deep, rich greens of the trees contrast dramatically with the lighter greens of the ferns. It's also very quiet here, except for the sounds of the woodland birds and critters. The caws of seagulls remind you that you're not only in the forest, but also very close to the ocean.

You might want to avoid the C loop. The sites are closer to each other, but more importantly, this is where the RVs come when they come to Seawall. If you have to, you can take a site in the C loop for a night or two, but do what you can to move into the D area or some of the more secluded sites in the A or B loop.

The D area has the walk-in tent sites. This is the stuff. This "village" of tent sites scattered throughout the forest is sublime. You park along a central loop, then walk into your site. The sites are anywhere from 20 feet to more than 100 feet from the parking area. Signs along the parking loop tell you which sites you're parking near.

These tent sites are all relatively uniform in size and character, and they are liberally sprinkled throughout the fairly thick forest of slender coniferous trees. The sites are moderately spacious—you'll be able to see a few of your neighbors, but there's not an obnoxious lack of privacy so much as a quiet sense of being covered by the forest canopy. The subcanopy here has an airy quality similar to that of the B loop. At night, the forest seems to close in around you and your campsite. It's very quiet here. All you'll hear are muffled conversations punctuated by the occasional snap of a campfire.

This community of tent sites is unlike anything I've seen at any other campground. The sense of solitude here is deep and complete. A network of walking paths just inside the woods leads you to all the sites, and little signposts at the intersections guide you to specific sites. It could get a bit confusing back here, so you'll definitely want to make sure you have a campground map handy.

The whole D area is phenomenal. A few sites are spread farther out than others, but overall the character of the forest, the site spaciousness, and the solitude are relatively similar throughout. Anywhere within the D area is a great place to spend a few nights in a tent.

You can tell the veteran D-area campers (like the veteran campers at Grout Pond in Vermont) because they arrive with some sort of wheeled cart or wagon to haul in their gear. Whether you have wheels or not, it's well worth the extra effort to get yourself to one of these sites within the D-area tent village in the woods. You'll be rewarded with refreshing wilderness solitude.

MAP

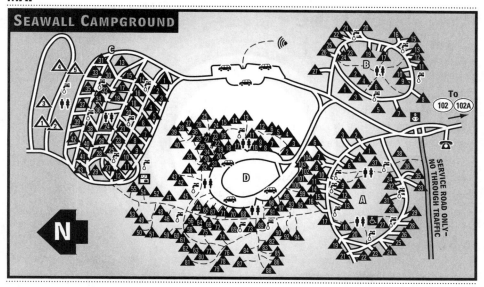

GETTING THERE

Follow ME 3 onto Mount Desert Island. Bear right onto ME 102/198 toward Southwest Harbor. Stay on ME 102. Follow ME 102 to ME 102A. Stay on ME 102A and follow the signs to the campground.

GPS COORDINATES

N44° 14.436285'
W68° 18.244908'

13 WARREN ISLAND STATE PARK

WHEN YOU JOURNEY TO WARREN ISLAND, you'll see the truth in the statement "half the fun is getting there." Warren Island is, after all, an island— you can't drive there, you can't hike there, and you certainly can't park an RV there. You *can* get there by kayak or canoe, one placid paddle stroke at a time. You can also get there by motorboat or sailboat, but most of the people you'll see camped out on Warren Island arrive by sea kayak.

Most of the island's campsites are spread along the shore; the rest are located toward the center of the island. There are six primitive tent sites, three group sites, and three Appalachian Mountain Club–style lean-tos. The day-use picnic sites and the overnight camping sites are available by reservation or a first-come, first-served basis. The only site you can't reserve is site 12, on the western shore of the island. The number and configuration of the sites does change, so please check when you make reservations.

The island is covered in a dense green spruce forest. Island camping in general, and certainly a night spent camping on Warren Island, is an olfactory experience. At any moment, in any breath, you can smell the crisp aroma of the spruce forest and the rich, heady scents of the sea.

It's funny to look down as you're walking along the Island Trail and see bits of shell mixed in with the pine needles and fallen leaves on the forest floor. The Island Trail is a walking trail that essentially circumnavigates the 70-acre island and brings you past most of the sites.

As you start to set up your camping gear, you'll notice a 5-gallon white bucket next to every fireplace and grill. It should be full of water. If it's not, be a good citizen and fill it up at the shore. This is Warren Island's volunteer fire department, and you're the firefighter. If your fire gets out of control, there's no calling 911, and

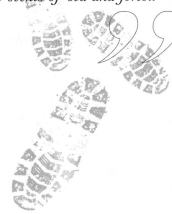

Warren Island is a slice of paradise. After an adventurous day of paddling on the ocean, you can relax by your campfire and enjoy the pristine view and the magnificent scents of sea and forest.

RATINGS

Beauty: ☆☆☆☆☆
Privacy: ☆☆☆☆☆
Spaciousness: ☆☆☆☆☆
Quiet: ☆☆☆☆☆
Security: ☆☆☆☆☆
Cleanliness: ☆☆☆☆☆

there's no truck on the island waiting to come douse the flames. An out-of-control campfire could be lethal, and that scenario is a major concern for island-dwellers and Warren Island State Park's ranger. Be extra-cautious with your fire, and make sure that bucket is full and next to the hearth.

Warren Island has no camp store, and cutting down or otherwise damaging trees is strictly forbidden. The rangers leave small caches of firewood here and there for campers. Be frugal and conserve wood. Build a fire only as large as you need to cook, stay warm, and keep the fireside ambience in your site. You'll save wood, minimize the risk to Warren Island, and still have a fantastically peaceful evening. OK, end of sermon.

After reaching the island from whichever direction you approach, you can access it via the pier on the east side, facing the Islesboro ferry terminal. Just off the end of the pier is the ranger station and the day-use area, with grills and picnic tables. If you're just pulling in for the day, the fee is $1, which you pay at the "Iron Ranger" posted at the head of the pier.

Head out on the Island Trail to the north (or to the right as you look onto the island from the end of the pier) and you'll find the campsites. Site 1 is situated on a grassy area, close to the restrooms and the pier, on the island's eastern shore. This site is on the inland side of the Island Trail.

Site 2 is the first of the sites situated right on the water. This site is marvelously spacious and well secluded. You can see the narrow bay that separates Warren and Islesboro islands through the loosely spaced trees that define the site. This site has two picnic tables and a stone hearth.

KEY INFORMATION

ADDRESS:	P.O. Box 105
	Lincolnville, ME 04849
OPERATED BY:	Maine Department of Conservation, Bureau of Parks and Lands
INFORMATION:	207-446-7090 or 207-941-4014 (off-season)
OPEN:	May 15–Sept. 15
SITES:	9 tent sites, 3 group sites, 3 lean-tos
EACH SITE:	Picnic table, stone hearth, fire bucket
ASSIGNMENT:	First-come, first-served or by reservation: 800-332-1501 (out of state), 207-624-9950 (in state), campwithme.com (additional $2 fee per site per night for reservations)
REGISTRATION:	At ranger station as you enter campground; check in after 1 p.m., check out by 11 a.m.
FACILITIES:	Pit toilets, water spigots, pier and moorings
PARKING:	Pull your kayak up on the beach!
FEE:	Maine residents, $14; nonresidents, $24; day-use fee, $1
RESTRICTIONS:	*Pets:* On leash only
	Fires: In established fire rings only
	Alcohol: Not allowed
	Vehicles: No vehicles on the island
	Other: Cutting or damaging trees is prohibited; campers must carry out all trash; no dishwashing at water spigots; quiet hours 10 p.m.–7 a.m., 14-day maximum stay

Deep in the woods on the forest side of the trail, site 3 is secluded and private. The inland sites at Warren Island are indeed lovely. But this is an island, so you'll probably be tempted to try to secure a waterfront site. It's well worth a little extra effort or wait.

The next oceanfront site is site 4, which is spacious and open, with cool breezes blowing off the ocean along with dramatic views of the bay. You can pull your kayaks right up to the edge of the site. If you arrive by a larger boat or don't paddle right up to the campsite, wheeled carts are available for hauling your gear from the pier.

Keep heading up the trail past sites 3 and 4, and you'll come to the North Shelter, one of the island's lean-tos. It's set in an open grove of birch and spruce trees, and it looks out over Penobscot Bay to the north. Its location perfectly blends a woodland setting and proximity to the island's shoreline.

The remaining inland sites are 8, 9, and 10. These group sites are set in a grassy field and among a grove of mixed forest in the center of the island. To reach them, take the short hiking trail that leads straight from the pier (heading west) and past the ranger station on the left. There are remnants from the foundation of a historic mansion out here. A water pump lies between sites 8 and 9, within the stone piles that suggest that a mansion stood here more than 80 years ago.

This mansion must have been quite a sight. It was once the property of William Folwell, a wool manufacturer from Philadelphia who purchased the land in 1899. At $75,000 (in turn-of-the-century dollars), it was believed to be one of the most expensive log cabins ever built in New England. The elegantly appointed "cabin" had 22 rooms, including a massive living room, dining room, and kitchen. Sadly, the structure burned to the ground in 1919.

Beyond sites 8 and 9 and the remnants of the Folwell mansion, site 10 is off in its own little field. The trio of inland sites is quite open and extraordinarily spacious. They offer less privacy than do the shoreline sites, and lack ocean views, but they are still beautiful. The breezes, the scent of the ocean, and the melancholy cry of the seagulls will remind you you're on an island.

Site 6 is way down on the Penobscot Bay (west) side of the island. Follow a short hiking trail from the open area near sites 8 and 9, and you'll find the shelter, which faces an absolutely priceless bay view.

Site 7 is down toward the southern end of the island. You can pull up to the pier on the east side and cart your gear down, or spot the site from the water and paddle right up to it. Not surprisingly, I prefer the second option.

This site has the most complete and deep sense of seclusion of any campsite in New England. You're at least 100 feet from your nearest neighbor, and all you can see are the woods and the bay. Two picnic tables and makeshift log benches sit by the fireplace at site 7. Set within a moderately spaced grove of spruce and other deciduous trees, it's quite open from above, so plenty of sunlight and moonlight filter in.

More often than not, a nice breeze wafts through the island, but on those still days, or during the morning and evening lull, the bugs can be ferocious. There is simply no escape. Think ahead and be prepared. Bring a head net and some of your favorite bug repellent.

Despite my earlier reverie about peaceful paddle strokes, the crossing from Camden or Lincolnville to Warren Island is wide open across more than 3 miles of Penobscot Bay. I've

MAP

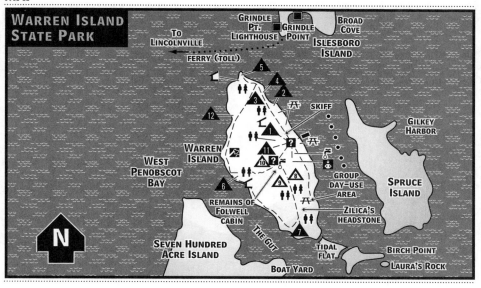

WARREN ISLAND STATE PARK

To LINCOLNVILLE
FERRY (TOLL)

GRINDLE PT. LIGHTHOUSE
GRINDLE POINT
BROAD COVE
ISLESBORO ISLAND

SKIFF
GILKEY HARBOR
WARREN ISLAND
WEST PENOBSCOT BAY
GROUP DAY-USE AREA
SPRUCE ISLAND
REMAINS OF FOLWELL CABIN
ZILICA'S HEADSTONE

N

SEVEN HUNDRED ACRE ISLAND
THE GUT
BOAT YARD
TIDAL FLAT
BIRCH POINT
LAURA'S ROCK

GETTING THERE

Drop your kayak in at Camden Harbor, Lincolnville Beach, or Ducktrap Harbor, and paddle east toward Islesboro. Warren Island is just southwest of the Islesboro ferry terminal.

GPS COORDINATES

N44° 16.436377'
W68° 56.620224'

crossed the bay when it was still as glass. I've also crossed it with clenched teeth, white knuckles, and the bow of my kayak slicing into the oncoming swells like a broadsword. Penobscot Bay is big water—exercise all sorts of caution. Don't paddle to Warren Island on your first kayak camping trip, or your second for that matter. Plan your trip carefully with respect to the winds, the tides, and the weather. If you're at all hesitant, wait for better weather or hire one of the area's registered guides.

If you do go over by yourself and get in a jam so you don't feel comfortable paddling back, paddle over to the ferry terminal on nearby Islesboro and see if you can hop on the ferry, which leaves Islesboro every hour on the half-hour. A round-trip adult ticket is $10, the rate for kids ages 5 to 11 is $4.75, and kids younger than 5 ride free.

A trip to Warren Island is one you'll remember for a long time to come. The combination of paddling or boating there, exploring the island, falling asleep to the delightful rustling of sea breeze in the pines, and waking up to the panorama of Penobscot Bay completes a mystical experience.

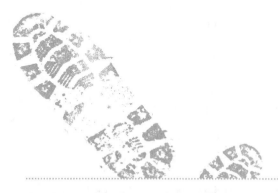

NEW HAMPSHIRE

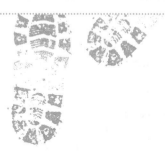

14
BEAR BROOK
STATE PARK

Allenstown

BEAR BROOK STATE PARK IS ENORMOUS—it's the largest state park in New Hampshire. Its size (the entire park spans more than 10,000 acres) and the myriad outdoor activities available here make this as much a destination as a place to set up camp. On the long road leading through the park and to the campground, I was convinced I had missed it. If you get this sensation, keep on going, because you're almost there. You'll come to another BEAR BROOK STATE PARK sign that points the way into the campground. The last stretch is a beautiful ride through a stately forest of pine and spruce trees that are at least 100 feet tall.

Bear Brook State Park has a massive network of trails, some of which pass right through the campground. You'll see trailheads for the Broken Boulder Trail and the Pitch Pine Trail on the last section of the campground road. Both of these trails eventually lead to Smith Pond.

The first loop within the campground (with sites 1 and up) is set beneath an open forest with very little undergrowth. These sites don't offer a lot of privacy, but they are spacious and centrally located within the campground. They're also covered by a blanket of pine needles. This loop is near an open field with a baseball diamond. There is even a small playground with a slide and swings—nice if you're camping with kids. If you want to be near these parts of the campground, check out sites 35 and 36, which are close to the baseball field.

Past the field, sites are tucked into the woods on the stretch of the campground road leading down to the small beach area on Beaver Pond. Sites 22 through 24 are nicely secluded and close to the pond. Of the other sites near the pond, site 31A is nice, as it's on the end of a short road jutting off the main campground road.

The beach at Beaver Pond is a great spot to spend an afternoon. You can paddle, fish, or just sit in the sand.

> *Bear Brook State Park has some great spots to camp in while you explore the rest of the park on foot, on a bike, or in a canoe.*

RATINGS

Beauty: ✩ ✩ ✩ ✩
Privacy: ✩ ✩ ✩ ✩
Spaciousness: ✩ ✩ ✩ ✩
Quiet: ✩ ✩ ✩
Security: ✩ ✩ ✩ ✩
Cleanliness: ✩ ✩ ✩ ✩

KEY INFORMATION

ADDRESS: 157 Deerfield Rd. Allenstown, NH 03275

OPERATED BY: New Hampshire Division of Parks and Recreation

INFORMATION: 603-485-9869 (campground office) or 603-485-9874 (park office)

OPEN: Memorial Day–Columbus Day

SITES: 99

EACH SITE: Fire ring, picnic table

ASSIGNMENT: First-come, first-served or by reservation: 877-647-2757, 603-271-3628, nhstateparks.org, or reserveamerica.com

REGISTRATION: At campground headquarters

FACILITIES: Flush toilets, showers, laundry, camp store, boat and canoe rentals, archery, nature center

PARKING: At sites

FEE: $23–$25

RESTRICTIONS: *Pets:* Dogs on leash only
Fires: In fire rings only
Alcohol: At sites only
Vehicles: Parking at campsites only, maximum 2 vehicles per site
Other: Reservations require 2-night minimum stay; check in 1–8 p.m., check out by noon; quiet hours 10 p.m.–7 a.m.

Being out in the deep woods and far from the ocean, this beach has no seashells—only pinecones! You don't have to worry about finding anything else in the sand either: no glass bottles, pets, or horses are allowed on the beach. The Beaver Pond trailhead is at the far end of the beach. This trail circumnavigates the pond, coming back in through the campground. From a small dock toward the end of the beach, you can launch kayak or canoe adventures.

As you head back toward the main part of the campground, sites 40 and 41 are quite spacious, although they're close to the headquarters and set within the open forest that covers most of the central campground loop. Like the lower-numbered sites, these are also blanketed with pine needles.

Site 55 is excellent; it's one of the more secluded at Bear Brook. A short perimeter of pines stands around the border as if guarding the site. Its neighbor, site 56, is also nicely isolated.

If you set up camp at site 64, you'll be able to pick up the Beaver Pond Trail right next to your campsite. Site 65 is off on its own, with a view of the pond through the loosely spaced forest that divides the campsites from the shores of the pond in this section of the campground.

Farther back on the campground loop road and away from the campground headquarters, you'll find site 94, another of Bear Brook's better choices. It's a spacious site set off on a small loop heading away from the pond. There is open forest both on the far side and overhead, so a lot of sunlight reaches it—you'll have a nice view of the night sky, too. There's also a self-guided nature trail adjacent.

Site 95 is truly secluded, at the end of a short spur leading off the main campground road. It has its own little cul-de-sac right in front of the site, so it's extremely spacious. It's set up against a small embankment and nestled within a grove of mixed hardwoods and conifers. Just outside the site to the left, a break in the forest gives you access to the pond. There's no beach here, but there's plenty of room to launch a canoe or kayak. This site is also near a trailhead that leads out of the campground.

MAP

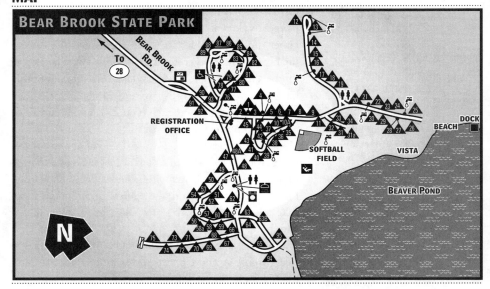

Site 75 is another secluded spot, at another end of the campground loop road and right on a dirt road leading out of the campground proper. Overall, sites 46 through 75 are more secluded than those in the rest of the campground. Some of these are much more spacious, and a few are positively perfect. The shower and laundry facilities are also within this group.

A special pond just for fly-fishing sits near the beginning of the road winding in toward the campground. The season runs from the fourth Saturday in April through October 15, and there's a limit of two brook trout per day. The park also boasts two archery ranges (apparently the only ones within the New Hampshire state-park system). For information on fishing licenses, see Appendix C, page 232.

If hiking, mountain biking, and paddling are more your speed, there's plenty of room for those as well. Many trails wind through Bear Brook State Park—more than 40 miles' worth—so you'll have to spend a lot of time here before you cross the same trail twice.

GETTING THERE

Take I-93 north through Manchester to the exit for NH 28 and NH 3 north. In Suncook, take NH 28 toward Allenstown. Turn right on Bear Brook Road.

GPS COORDINATES

N43° 6.942701'
W71° 19.694417'

15
BIG ROCK
CAMPGROUND

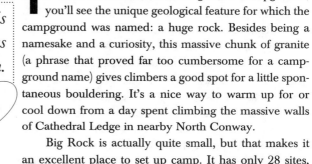

> *You'll know how this campground got its name as soon as you pull in.*

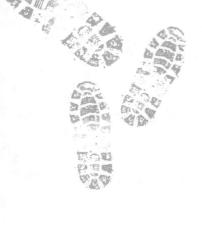

THE MOMENT YOU PULL INTO Big Rock Campground, you'll see the unique geological feature for which the campground was named: a huge rock. Besides being a namesake and a curiosity, this massive chunk of granite (a phrase that proved far too cumbersome for a campground name) gives climbers a good spot for a little spontaneous bouldering. It's a nice way to warm up for or cool down from a day spent climbing the massive walls of Cathedral Ledge in nearby North Conway.

Big Rock is actually quite small, but that makes it an excellent place to set up camp. It has only 28 sites, many of which have a decent amount of space and some privacy. If you've come camping with a group or need several sites, try to secure something in the range of sites 23 through 28. There's a small central parking area, so you'll have to haul in your gear, but not too far. These sites sit atop the small hill around which the campground is situated, isolating them from the rest of the campground, if not from each other. A restroom is right down the access road.

Other prime tent spots within Big Rock are sites 7, 8, 9, 12, and 13 through 18. All are on the same loop (the main loop of the campground). The forest here is a bit thicker than the open woods of nearby Hancock Campground (see page 86). It's a mixed forest of coniferous and deciduous trees, so at the height of summer the dense woods separate the sites as well.

I especially like the fact that this is such a small campground. Yes, it fills up quickly as a result, but if you get here early enough and secure a spot, you can rest assured that you'll have peaceful, quiet nights in the woods. Big Rock is only the second campground you'll come across as you travel east on Kancamagus Highway (or "The Kanc," as this delightful stretch of road is known to the locals and regulars), so it's still fairly close to Lincoln.

RATINGS

Beauty: ✪ ✪ ✪ ✪
Privacy: ✪ ✪ ✪ ✪
Spaciousness: ✪ ✪ ✪ ✪
Quiet: ✪ ✪ ✪ ✪ ✪
Security: ✪ ✪ ✪ ✪
Cleanliness: ✪ ✪ ✪ ✪

Big Rock is a great spot from which to launch your outdoor adventures, being a short drive or walk from some prime hikes and sights along The Kanc. Right across the road runs the Hancock Branch of the Pemigewasset. Stroll over there with a fishing rod or a towel, depending on your preference (for information on fishing licenses, see Appendix C, page 232).

Several hiking trails lie just a stone's throw down The Kanc. Turn left out of the campground, heading toward Conway, and you'll soon come to trailheads for the East Pond Trail and the Hancock Notch Trail. This trail follows the North Fork of the Pemigewasset for a while, then bears east toward Mount Huntington, Hancock Notch, and the Sawyer Pond Scenic Area. It would be a fairly sturdy hike from the Hancock Notch trailhead all the way to Sawyer Pond, so bring plenty of food and water if you're coming this way.

Across The Kanc from these trailheads is the Greeley Ponds Trail, which leads to the Greeley Ponds Scenic Area. If you've hiked in this far and still want to explore, the Mount Osceola Trail leads you up to East Peak, West Peak, and Mount Osceola. You'll also be able to sneak occasional views of Mount Kancamagus to the east.

It can sometimes be a challenge to secure one of the prime tent spots at Big Rock, because it's one of the first campgrounds to fill during the busy summer weekends. Even if you've come to The Kanc at the height of the season, it's well worth your time to take a swing through Big Rock just in case a spot is open.

Who knows what the campground might have been called had a careless glacier not casually dropped that massive boulder near the entrance several million years ago? On the other hand, who cares? Big Rock is small and cozy, and that makes it an ideally sized campground and a great spot to pitch a tent.

KEY INFORMATION

ADDRESS: Kancamagus Hwy. Lincoln, NH 03818

OPERATED BY: U.S. Forest Service, Pro Sport, Inc.

INFORMATION: Saco Ranger Station, 33 Kancamagus Hwy. (RFD 1, Box 94), Conway, NH 03818; 603-447-5448, icampnh.com

OPEN: Mid-May–mid-Oct.

SITES: 28

EACH SITE: Fire ring, picnic table

ASSIGNMENT: First-come, first-served

REGISTRATION: Select site, then pay at self-service fee station

FACILITIES: Vault toilets

PARKING: At sites

FEE: $20 for 1 vehicle, $5 for extra vehicle

RESTRICTIONS: *Pets:* Dogs on leash only
Fires: In fire rings only
Alcohol: At sites only
Vehicles: Maximum 2 per site
Other: Maximum 8 people per site; 14-day maximum stay

MAP

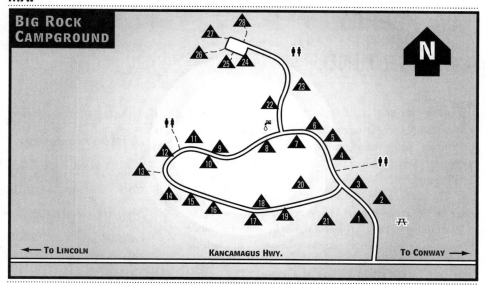

BIG ROCK CAMPGROUND

← To Lincoln   KANCAMAGUS HWY.   To Conway →

GETTING THERE

From Lincoln, follow
Kancamagus Highway to
Big Rock Campground,
on the left. From Conway,
follow Kancamagus
Highway to Big Rock
Campground, on the right.

GPS COORDINATES

N44° 2.819080'
W71° 33.566859'

16
BLACKBERRY CROSSING CAMPGROUND

THERE MAY BE just six sites set aside for tent camping at Blackberry Crossing Campground, but its character, history, and location on Kancamagus Highway make a trip here time well spent. It's another of the area's fairly small campgrounds, about the same size as Big Rock.

The six tent sites are in a small field on the eastern edge of the campground. They are tent-only owing to the fact that you have to lug your gear in a short distance from the parking area for this loop. Sites 21 through 26 are at the woods' edge around a central clearing about one-quarter the size of a football field. The open space between these tent sites adds a community flavor to this part of the campground. On crystal-clear, jet-black New England nights, you'll be thankful that you're far from any light pollution that might interfere with stargazing. The break in the trees over the field affords magnificent views of the skies. Keep an eye to the sky if you're there in mid-August, and you could catch the Perseid meteor showers.

During daylight hours, the field is a great spot for a quick game of Frisbee or a group picnic. It's also a great space to let the kids run around in and blow off steam while you kick back in the sun—or in the shade of the birch, pine, and mixed deciduous forest. Either way, you'll still have a full view of your gang. It's also just 6 miles west of Conway if you need anything, from groceries to a hot pizza.

Blackberry Crossing looks quite different than it did 70-something years ago. Nearly 200 men lived and worked here between 1935 and 1941 as part of President Roosevelt's "Tree Army." Blackberry Crossing was home to Company 1177 of the Civilian Conservation Corps, which cut most of the trails in and around the White Mountains that we still enjoy today.

Besides preserving and providing access to wilderness, the CCC employed men during the depths of the

> *Blackberry Crossing is rich in history, with tall stone hearths remaining from its days as a Civilian Conservation Corps camp.*

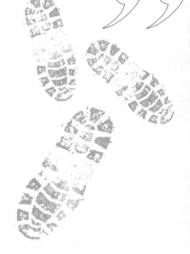

RATINGS

Beauty: ✩ ✩ ✩ ✩
Privacy: ✩ ✩ ✩
Spaciousness: ✩ ✩ ✩ ✩
Quiet: ✩ ✩ ✩
Security: ✩ ✩ ✩ ✩
Cleanliness: ✩ ✩ ✩ ✩

ADDRESS:	Kancamagus Hwy. Albany, NH 03818
OPERATED BY:	U.S. Forest Service, Pro Sport, Inc.
INFORMATION:	Saco Ranger Station, 33 Kancamagus Hwy. (RFD 1, Box 94), Conway, NH 03818; 603-447-5448, icampnh.com
OPEN:	April–Nov.
SITES:	26
EACH SITE:	Fire ring, picnic table
ASSIGNMENT:	First-come, first-served
REGISTRATION:	Select site, then pay at self-service fee station
FACILITIES:	Vault toilets, hand pump for water
PARKING:	At sites; separate parking area for tent loop
FEE:	$20 for 1 vehicle, $5 for extra vehicle
RESTRICTIONS:	*Pets:* **Dogs on leash only** *Fires:* **In fire rings only** *Alcohol:* **At sites only** *Vehicles:* **Maximum 2 per site** *Other:* **Maximum 8 people per site; 14-day maximum stay**

Great Depression. There are still a few remnants of Blackberry Crossing's days as a CCC encampment, most notably two large stone hearths—one right by site 20 and the other between sites 8 and 9. These are all that remain of the camp's original headquarters and recreation hall.

The sites in the tent loop are obviously the best for tent camping, but if you've come with a large group or several families and that loop is already occupied, you could also look into sites 7, 9 and 11. These are on the outside of the central loop. You'll be close to one of the beautiful old stone hearths and a historic marker with photos of the camp in its heyday. These sites are wide open, but they're set amid a lovely grove of birch trees. Sites 14 and 15, roughly between the central loop and the tent-only loop, are also off on their own.

Whether you've come to Blackberry Crossing to camp for one night or for a whole week, don't miss Rocky Gorge. Visit it by heading out of the campground and taking a left. A series of natural pools and rock baths leads to a fairly steep and wild waterfall. The Swift River gets narrow and speeds through the gorge here. A footbridge leads right over the waterfall, so you can get a spectacular view of the show beneath.

Follow the footbridge to the trail on the opposite side of the river, and a short hike will lead you to the placid, quiet Falls Pond. There's a hiking trail that leads all the way around the pond as well.

Blackberry Crossing Campground is directly opposite Covered Bridge Campground (see next profile), which is kind of amusing. If you're camping with a large group or have a particular affinity for historic sites, Blackberry Crossing is definitely worth a look. If it's just you and a friend, you might want to head across the road to Covered Bridge.

MAP

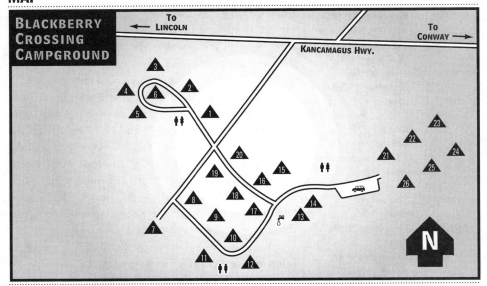

BLACKBERRY CROSSING CAMPGROUND

To ← LINCOLN

To CONWAY →

KANCAMAGUS HWY.

N

GETTING THERE

From Lincoln, follow Kancamagus Highway to Blackberry Crossing Campground, on your right. From Conway, follow Kancamagus Highway to Blackberry Crossing Campground, on your left and across the street from Covered Bridge Campground.

GPS COORDINATES

N43° 59.749804'
W71° 13.516803'

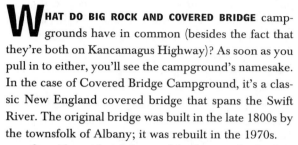

> *The campground's proximity to a massive rock garden and two trailheads makes Covered Bridge a great spot for hikers.*

WHAT DO BIG ROCK AND COVERED BRIDGE campgrounds have in common (besides the fact that they're both on Kancamagus Highway)? As soon as you pull in to either, you'll see the campground's namesake. In the case of Covered Bridge Campground, it's a classic New England covered bridge that spans the Swift River. The original bridge was built in the late 1800s by the townsfolk of Albany; it was rebuilt in the 1970s.

On either side of the road leading to the bridge, huge timbers span the road at a 7-foot, 9-inch height to ensure that "adventurous" RV or camper owners don't try to drive through the bridge. Effective in preserving this historic covered bridge, the timbers also help keep the larger RVs out of Covered Bridge Campground. (You can get into the campground from the Dugway Road, 6 miles west of Conway . . . but don't tell anyone in an RV!)

Coming into the campground from the Kancamagus, you'll pass under the RV trap with ease, traverse the covered bridge (keep an eye out for pedestrians—covered bridges throughout New England always draw camera-toting crowds), and bear right on Dugway Road. The campground is on the left, about 0.5 mile down the road. As soon as you cross the bridge and bear right, you'll see the parking area and trailhead for the Boulder Loop Trail on the right. Make a mental note to walk back later for a quick hike.

Covered Bridge Campground is moderate in size, with 49 sites. There are no tent-only sites, but some practical landscape considerations make this a great campground for a night in the nylon. As soon as you pull into the campground, keep bearing left. This will bring you to the small dead-end loop with sites 25 through 27. These are great sites, set off on their own amid the fairly dense, mostly coniferous forest. Just outside this loop is site 24, which is set against a garden of massive

RATINGS

Beauty: ✿ ✿ ✿ ✿ ✿
Privacy: ✿ ✿ ✿ ✿
Spaciousness: ✿ ✿ ✿ ✿
Quiet: ✿ ✿ ✿ ✿ ✿
Security: ✿ ✿ ✿ ✿
Cleanliness: ✿ ✿ ✿ ✿ ✿

boulders—no doubt spilled over from the aptly named Boulder Loop Trail.

Generally speaking, the outer-loop sites are the best. If you're fortunate enough, you'll be able to score one of the northernmost sites set off on their own platforms, which means you have to lug your tent and other gear up a short incline. If you're on the southern end of the loop, you might be somewhere near an RV, but the sites are spacious and distant enough to provide solitude.

The northern-loop sites that make up the prime tent spots at Covered Bridge are 17, 19, 41, 43, 45, 47, and 49. These sites back up to a massive cliff that rises just behind the campground. During the summer, the forest may be too dense for you to fully appreciate this grand formation, which is part of the granite pile left by the glaciers that scraped through here thousands of years ago.

One other way to appreciate the geologic uniqueness of this area is to head down Dugway Road, back toward the covered bridge, and take a spin around the Boulder Loop Trail. The trail will take you up and around the side of this cliff and through a delightful garden of huge boulders. The beginning of this trail resembles a massive stone staircase. You almost expect it to lead to a giant's castle. The glaciers inadvertently created a hiker's playground here, but watch your step: it's quite easy to twist an ankle when hiking and bounding through the boulders.

Another nice trailhead right near the campground is the Lower Nanamocomuck Ski Trail, just past the covered bridge coming from the campground. This makes for a fairly level hike during the spring, summer, and fall and a dramatic backcountry-skiing or snowshoeing trek in the winter. While Covered Bridge Campground isn't open during the winter, Hancock Campground (see page 86) is open year-round.

One historical aspect of Covered Bridge can add a bit of spice to your ghost stories around the campfire: As soon as you enter the campground, there's a small, fenced-off burial plot. After dinner, stroll down to the burial site, make sure no one from the Lane family (the name on the headstone) is up and about, then go whip up a couple of ghoulish tales with a local connection!

ADDRESS:	Dugway Rd.. Albany, NH 03818
OPERATED BY:	U.S. Forest Service, Pro Sport, Inc.
INFORMATION:	Saco Ranger Station, 33 Kancamagus Hwy. (RFD 1, Box 94), Conway, NH 03818; 603-447-5448, icampnh.com
OPEN:	Mid-May–mid-Oct.
SITES:	49
EACH SITE:	Fire ring, picnic table
ASSIGNMENT:	First-come, first-served; sites 9–17, 29–37, 39–47 by reservation Memorial Day–Columbus Day: 877-444-6777, recreation.gov
REGISTRATION:	Select a site, then pay at self-service fee station
FACILITIES:	Vault toilets near fishing pier on Swift River
PARKING:	At sites
FEE:	$20 for 1 vehicle, $5 for extra vehicle
RESTRICTIONS:	*Pets:* Dogs on leash only *Fires:* In fire rings only *Alcohol:* At sites only *Vehicles:* Maximum 2 per site *Other:* Maximum 8 people per site; 14-day maximum stay

MAP

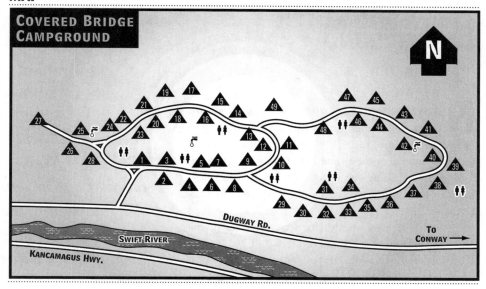

GETTING THERE

From Lincoln, follow
Kancamagus Highway to
Covered Bridge Camp-
ground, to your left on Dugway Road, across the covered
bridge and opposite Blackberry Crossing Campground.
From Conway, follow Kan-
camagus Highway to Cov-
ered Bridge Campground, on
your right on Dugway Road,
across the covered bridge
and opposite Blackberry
Crossing Campground.

GPS COORDINATES

N44° 0.199800'
W71° 13.933203'

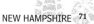

18
CRAWFORD NOTCH CAMPGROUND

NESTLED WITHIN THE WILDERNESS of Crawford Notch, the campground of the same name is a perfectly peaceful spot to pitch your tent—whether you've come to this part of the state for the climbing, hiking, fishing, or just sitting and watching the Saco River flow by. (For information on fishing licenses, see Appendix C, page 232.)

Note: This area was hit hard by flooding in the aftermath of Hurricane Irene in the fall of 2011. Consequently, the campground has undergone quite a bit of reconfiguring. Some of these efforts may be continuing as of this writing, so call (603-374-2779), check the website (**crawfordnotchcamping.com**), and/or consult the current map (see page 74) before you go. Some advance planning will be worth it to ensure that you get the site you want.

Crawford Notch is meticulously maintained, with a clean, sandy surface on the roads throughout the campground and on the individual sites. A dense forest, mostly young maples and beech, covers the campground. The deciduous trees display a brilliant, shimmering-green character, especially when their leaves are backlit by the sun. This dense forest also gives most of the sites a marvelous sense of seclusion. Many of the sites here are on or near the shores of the Saco River; these are by far the most spectacular.

The first sites you'll see as you drive into the campground are the cabins and RV sites with hookups. These sites are also close to the road and are fairly open to each other. Considering the magical quality of some of the riverside hike-in spots here, you should keep driving to find the primo sites.

As you drive a bit deeper into the campground, sites 38 and 39 are carved out of the beech forest. They're near the river but not right on the riverbanks. Continuing on down the campground road toward the riverbanks, you'll

> *Deep in the wilderness of Crawford Notch, campsites here are carved out of dense forest, and many are perched on the banks of the Saco River.*

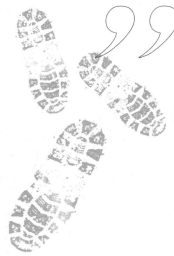

RATINGS

Beauty: ☆ ☆ ☆ ☆ ☆
Privacy: ☆ ☆ ☆ ☆
Spaciousness: ☆ ☆ ☆ ☆
Quiet: ☆ ☆ ☆ ☆
Security: ☆ ☆ ☆ ☆
Cleanliness: ☆ ☆ ☆ ☆ ☆

KEY INFORMATION

ADDRESS: US 302
Harts Location,
NH 03812

OPERATED BY: Crawford Notch
General Store and
Campground

INFORMATION: 603-374-2779,
crawfordnotch
camping.com

OPEN: Mid-May–mid-Oct.

SITES: 74

EACH SITE: Fire ring or stone
hearth, picnic table

ASSIGNMENT: First-come, first-
served; by reserva-
tion (recommended
in July and August
or during foliage
season, late Sept.–
early Oct.)

REGISTRATION: At campground
office and store
located on US 302

FACILITIES: Portable toilets,
shower building,
water spigots

PARKING: At campsites or
in shared parking
areas

FEE: $30–$38 (depend-
ing on location
of site)

RESTRICTIONS: *Pets:* Dogs on
leash only
Fires: At fire rings
only
Alcohol: At sites
Vehicles: Maximum
1 per site
Other: Check in 1–
9 p.m., quiet hours
10 p.m.–7 a.m.;
check out by 11 a.m.

come to sites 1 through 4 and sites 43, 44, and 45—argu-ably the best sites at Crawford Notch. These riverside sites may not afford as much seclusion as the sites in the deep woods, but the views of the cliffs are dramatic, and you'll fall asleep to the sounds of the Saco meandering past your tent.

Moving down the river, heading south, you'll find sites 47 and 48 and sites 53 and 52. All but site 52 are hike-in sites. Off to the other side of that cul-de-sac are a handful of other riverside sites. Sites 55, 55A, 55B, and 55C are all a short hike from the campground road. That distance, plus the slightly more dense forest here, gives these sites a beautiful sense of seclusion. And again, they're right on the Saco River.

Deeper into the forest on this side, you'll find sites 104 through 106. All three are spectacularly secluded. Site 104 lies deeper in the woods, but sites 105 and 106 are riverside. Off the farthest spur on the campground road are sites 95 through 103. All are good-sized and very nicely secluded. They're not hike-in sites, but because they're set off the road a bit, they offer an enhanced sense of privacy.

The hike-in sites along the Saco River are dramati-cally beautiful. They are incredibly remote-feeling yet easily accessible, perched as they are along or near the shores of the Saco. The drive-in sites are easier to get into to unload your gear, but the hike-in sites offer a sense of wilderness and seclusion that astounds me. I always prefer these types of sites, even if it means a little extra effort hauling gear.

Back toward the center of the campground, along the campground road, are sites 56 through 63. Site 56 also has a short hike in. It's secluded but somewhat small. Site 59 is nicely secluded, with a bit of a hike in. You'll also have a short hike to site 62, but it's huge and very private. This would be an excellent site for a larger group. There's a short hike into site 61 as well. Although this site is much smaller, it's isolated from the road and from neighboring sites.

Site 63 is not only very spacious but also has its own tent platform, so you're guaranteed a level, dry space upon which to pitch your tent. Sites 63A and 64 are both secluded and set against Beaver Pond.

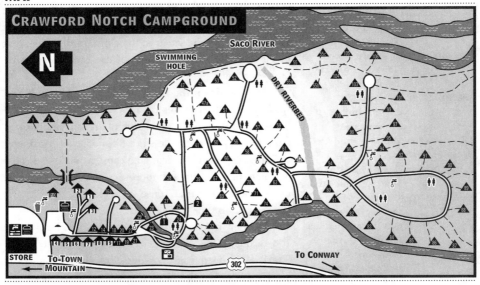

CRAWFORD NOTCH CAMPGROUND

SACO RIVER

SWIMMING HOLE

DRY RIVERBED

STORE

To-Town MOUNTAIN

TO CONWAY

302

Sites 65 through 71 are all drive-in sites situated on a short spur off the primary campground road. Sites 65 and 66 are both moderate in size, and they are very secluded from each other and from the other sites on this part of the loop. The locations are staggered on either side of the road, so your site here won't be open to the neighboring one across the way. Plus, these sites are all carved from a dense forest.

Site 68 is large, and it's peppered with slightly older beech and birch trees that provide a beautiful canopy of leaves. Site 69 is set well off the road and somewhat private, even though it's also close to the toilets. Sites 70 and 71 share a parking area, but there is enough forest separating the two sites that they also share a sense of deep-woods seclusion. Site 70 is framed by a bed of ferns that give it an almost primeval feeling. This site is a bit smaller than the others in this loop, but the scenic seclusion is well worth it. Site 71 is much larger.

The rest of the sites in this loop, 72 through 75, lie along a cul-de-sac at the end of the road. Sites 73 and 75 are especially close to the water, which makes them preferable.

GETTING THERE

From North Conway, follow US 302 north into Crawford Notch and White Mountain National Forest. The campground will be on your right, 13.5 miles past the intersection where NH 16 splits from US 302.

GPS COORDINATES

N44° 10.925682'
W71° 23.934753'

Another loop deeper into the campground hosts the sites in the 80s and low 90s. Along this loop, sites 88 through 93 are set into the deep woods and have a nice remote feel.

Crawford Notch is home to renowned climbing routes at Frankenstein Cliffs, hiking trails that wind past numerous waterfalls, and of course the Saco River. Whatever brings you to the area, Crawford Notch Campground is a scenic and secluded spot for setting up base camp.

19
DOLLY COPP
CAMPGROUND

Gorham

THE **WHITE MOUNTAIN NATIONAL FOREST** is a paradise for camping, hiking, biking, fly-fishing, canoeing, and nearly every other outdoor pursuit: it's "The Land of Many Uses," as the U.S. Forest Service signs proclaim. All those sound like pretty good uses to me, and I'm certainly not alone. During all four seasons, a steady flow of fun-hogs pours into the Mount Washington Valley. Don't be too dismayed if it seems like everyone else in the free world is heading north with you. Many also come for the indoor activities, like outlet shopping in North Conway.

You can escape some of the crowds who may not head any farther north than the outlets by heading farther north yourself, to Dolly Copp Campground. The campground is just north of Mount Washington and right off NH 16. Don't make the mistake of pulling in to the Dolly Copp picnic area—the campground is another mile up the road.

Dolly Copp is a good-sized campground, and it's not packed with sites. Instead, 173 sites are distributed in nine separate areas, between which there is plenty of room. You won't find any tent-specific areas within Dolly Copp, but there are a few areas where trailers aren't allowed. These loops are more secluded, densely forested, and perfect for pitching a tent. The only area that you would definitely want to avoid is the Big Meadow area, which includes sites 1 through 50. This area has most of the open sites where the land yachts come to drop anchor.

A respectful distance farther up the campground-access road is where you'll find the prime tent sites. Brook Loop is a great spot for tent campers. No trailers are allowed here. This loop includes sites 75 through 91. Within Brook Loop, sites 80 through 84 are in their own little mini-loop—perfect if you're camping with a large group. Even if some other folks are already camped out

> *Dolly Copp is like several small campgrounds rolled into one, with lots of cozy spots tucked into the dense forest.*

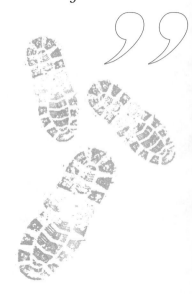

RATINGS

Beauty: ✿ ✿ ✿ ✿
Privacy: ✿ ✿ ✿ ✿
Spaciousness: ✿ ✿ ✿
Quiet: ✿ ✿ ✿ ✿
Security: ✿ ✿ ✿ ✿
Cleanliness: ✿ ✿ ✿ ✿

KEY INFORMATION

ADDRESS: NH 16
Gorham, NH 03581

OPERATED BY: U.S. Forest Service,
Pro Sport, Inc.

INFORMATION: Androscoggin
Ranger Station,
300 Glen Rd.,
Gorham, NH
03581; 603-466-
2713, icampnh.com

OPEN: Mid-May–mid-Oct.

SITES: 173

EACH SITE: Fire pit

ASSIGNMENT: First-come, first-
served; sites 1, 2,
4–12, 14, 28–33,
35–44, 46–50, 51,
53, 65–72, 75–77,
79, 85–91, 92–96a,
105–109, 121–123,
125–134, 136, 140–
149, 154, 155, 159,
160, 162–168 by
reservation Memo-
rial Day–Columbus
Day: 877-444-6777,
recreation.gov

REGISTRATION: At campground
headquarters

FACILITIES: Flush toilets, water

PARKING: At sites

FEE: $20 for 1 vehicle,
$5 for extra
vehicle

RESTRICTIONS: *Pets:* Dogs on
leash only
Fires: In fire
pits only; no
unattended fires
Alcohol: At sites only
Vehicles: Maximum
1 per site; trail-
ers prohibited in
Spruce Woods and
Brook Loop

in the 80-through-84 loop, you'll still be able to experi-ence solitude. From where you park your vehicle, you have to walk up to tent platforms for two of the sites within the loop, and down to a platform for another, so they are a bit more set off.

Spruce Woods is another great spot for tents. No trail-ers are allowed here, and the road is narrow and winding, so you're unlikely to see any large, self-contained camp-ers. The Spruce Woods Loop includes sites 51 through 72. As soon as you turn in to this loop, you'll feel as if you're driving deeper into the forest. The whole area is densely wooded with fir, pine, and spruce trees, giving it a nice sylvan atmosphere. The forest floor remains cool even on the sultriest summer day, and the sunlight filters down through the trees in fractured columns, adding a mystical air to the woods. Even if you have neighbors on both sides, you may not be able to see them. This is my favorite section of Dolly Copp.

The only drawback to the dense forest is that you won't have a very good view of the night sky for stargaz-ing. On a clear night, you can always take a short walk to an open area or even down to the banks of the Peabody River, which flows by just outside the campground.

There are several campground hosts who stay at the same well-marked sites throughout the season. The hosts are a good source of information on campground regu-lations, what to do in the area, and Rockwellian local lore, if you have a moment to chat. The rangers at Dolly Copp also run various visitor programs and interpretive walks during the season. If you've come to the White Mountains for some fly-fishing, you'll be able to find quite a few secluded fishing spots on either the Peabody River or the Moose River, which is just a bit farther north (for information on fishing licenses, see Appendix C, page 232).

Then there's the hiking. It's everywhere. Dolly Copp is a great place to set up your base camp if you've come to the White Mountains to hike Mount Washington, the rest of the Presidential Range, or anywhere within the White Mountain National Forest.

Along Kancamagus Highway and up NH 16 are numerous trailheads. You can find a hike that is long, short, steep, gradual—whatever suits your mood, your

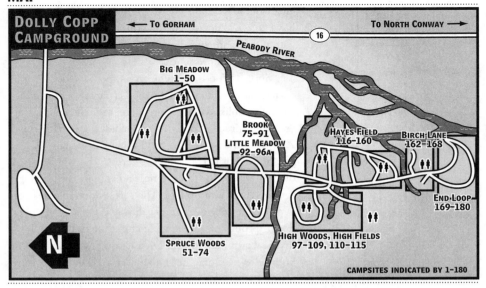

DOLLY COPP CAMPGROUND

← TO GORHAM   TO NORTH CONWAY →

16

PEABODY RIVER

BIG MEADOW
1–50

BROOK
75–91
LITTLE MEADOW
92–96A

HAYES FIELD
116–160

BIRCH LANE
162–168

END LOOP
169–180

SPRUCE WOODS
51–74

HIGH WOODS, HIGH FIELDS
97–109, 110–115

CAMPSITES INDICATED BY 1–180

N

energy level, or the amount of time you have before heading back to the real world.

As someone who skis Tuckerman Ravine every spring, I always find myself questioning my sanity when I get a good view of the Left Gully and the rest of the ravine without snow. It's almost unthinkable that people hike up there, much less ski down.

If you come to the Mount Washington area for winter activities such as mountaineering or ice-climbing and you want to camp, you won't be able to do so at Dolly Copp, which closes in mid-October. However, Barnes Field, which is off the access road leading into Dolly Copp, is open year-round for individual camping and for group camping in season by reservation only.

GETTING THERE

From North Conway, follow NH 16 north past the AMC Pinkham Notch Base Camp and the Mount Washington Auto Road. The campground will be on the left. From Gorham, follow NH 16 south to the campground, on your right. If you come to the Mount Washington Auto Road, you've gone too far.

GPS COORDINATES

N44° 20.159283'
W71° 12.592664'

20
DRY RIVER
CAMPGROUND

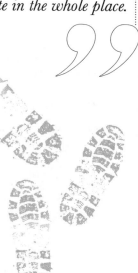

> *Dry River Campground is quiet and intimate. It's one of those campgrounds where there's really not a bad site in the whole place.*

DON'T GET CONFUSED as you drive up through Crawford Notch State Park. The state-park campground is called Dry River Campground. There's also a Crawford Notch Campground (see page 72), but that's a private campground across US 302. Both are excellent camping spots near some fantastic hiking and climbing routes.

Dry River is one of those campgrounds where there's not a bad site in the place. It's a small campground set within a moderately dense forest of mixed deciduous trees: maple, birch, and ash. All the campsites are very clean and spacious. The setting in Crawford Notch doesn't hurt one bit either. From your campsite, you're minutes from dramatically beautiful and challenging trails, world-class rock-climbing at Frankenstein Cliffs, and towering waterfalls. You won't run out of things to do or places to explore when staying here.

Most of the sites are spread out along a short loop that shoots off to the left as you enter the campground. Several sites lie down a short road running straight off to the right, but we'll get to those later. (*Note:* The campground may have undergone significant reconfiguration as of this writing, so check before you go: 603-374-2272, **nhstateparks.org,** or **reserveamerica.com.**)

A deep wilderness atmosphere pervades this campground. The trees open above most of the sites, which allows lots of light to filter down. Overall, Dry River's sites are laid out thoughtfully, both individually and in relation to one another. The sites aren't too densely packed together, and they fit in well with the forest's character.

The sites on the outside of the campground loop road provide the greatest seclusion and are also a bit larger than the others. You'll have plenty of room to spread out your tents and the rest of your gear, plus enough room to let the kids run around and tire themselves out.

There's also typically more forestation between sites here, which deepens the feeling of solitude. Sites 9, 11,

RATINGS

Beauty: ✰ ✰ ✰ ✰ ✰
Privacy: ✰ ✰ ✰ ✰
Spaciousness: ✰ ✰ ✰ ✰
Quiet: ✰ ✰ ✰
Security: ✰ ✰ ✰ ✰ ✰
Cleanliness: ✰ ✰ ✰ ✰

and 16 through 21, on the outside of the campground loop road, provide pleasant isolation and lots of space. Just past site 9 is a trailhead for a short path down to Dry River.

One of the prettiest sites here is site 16. It's set off the campground loop road, with lots of room between it and neighboring sites. It's also the site closest to Dry River. Between sites 18 and 19 are trails to the Dry River Connection. From the campground, it's 0.2 mile to Dry River, 2 miles to the Webster Cliff Trail, and 3 miles to the historic Willey House site.

Way off on its own, site 20 is another epic spot. It's incredibly spacious and surrounded by colossal deciduous trees with a few conifers mixed in, which gives the forest a diverse and interesting character.

There is still a decent sense of solitude to site 8, even though it's probably the most open site at Dry River, situated right where the campground loop reconnects with itself. Sites 4 through 7 and 22 through 24 lie along the campground road leading to the loop, but they are all well off the road.

Sites 27 through 31 are closer to US 302, but they are among the nicest sites I've seen. Situated along a short spur off the road, just off to the right as you enter the campground (even before the ranger station), these sites are spacious and spread out.

The only site to which I wouldn't immediately gravitate is site 31, which is set at the very end of this short road and opens directly to it, so anyone driving down the road would look like they're going to drive right into your site. Still, it's very spacious and otherwise isolated, so it's not that bad. The only other drawback—and this is very minor—is that these sites are closer to US 302. This can make for a bit of daytime road noise, but at night it's as silent as the rest of the White Mountains.

Opposite site 29 is a cluster of platform tent sites, numbers P1 through P6. Another platform site sits next to site 21, numbered P7. Newer than the previous numbered sites, these have platforms that ensure a solid surface for your tent.

The character of Dry River Campground mirrors that of its setting within Crawford Notch. There's a pleasant feel to the diverse forest and campground, and no matter where you end up, you'll be in an excellent spot.

KEY INFORMATION

ADDRESS: P.O. Box 177 US 302 Twin Mountain, NH 03595

OPERATED BY: New Hampshire Division of Parks and Recreation

INFORMATION: 603-374-2272

OPEN: Late April–early Dec.

SITES: 38

EACH SITE: Fire ring, picnic table

ASSIGNMENT: First-come, first-served or by reservation: 877-647-2757, 603-271-3628, nhstateparks .org, or reserve america.com

REGISTRATION: At campground headquarters

FACILITIES: Hot showers, pit toilets

PARKING: At sites

FEE: $23–$25

RESTRICTIONS: *Pets:* On leash only
Fires: In fire rings only
Alcohol: At sites only
Vehicles: Parking at campsites only
Other: Reservations require 2-night minimum stay; check in 1–8 p.m., check out by noon; quiet hours 10 p.m.–7 a.m.

MAP

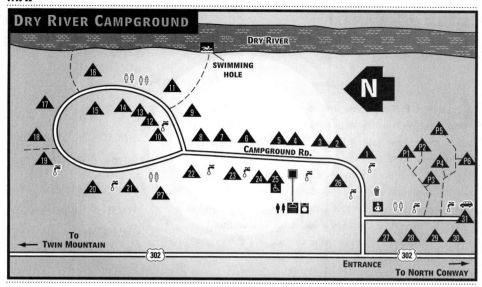

GETTING THERE

From North Conway and
Bartlett, continue north on
US 302 and look for signs for
the campground, on the right.

GPS COORDINATES

N44° 9.363177'
W71° 21.788728'

21
GILSON POND CAMPGROUND

GILSON POND is the first new campground in the New Hampshire state-park system in more than 40 years—pretty exciting stuff in the camping world. The summer of 2010 was the first season it was open. The original Monadnock State Park campground is still open, but it's available only for youth group camping during the regular season—when Gilson Pond Campground is open. Before Memorial Day and after Columbus Day, when Gilson Pond is closed for the season, the original MSP campground remains open for off-season and winter camping.

Gilson Pond Campground is indeed a gem through and through. It's clean and quiet, most of the sites provide the deep sense of solitude that I so enjoy, and the whole campground is still within range of the entire network of hiking trails at MSP. You could reach the summit of the 3,165-foot Mount Monadnock right from your campsite (following the Birchtoft Trail, which leaves the campground just below sites A17 and A18).

Sites A1 and A2 are spectacularly isolated, set off on their own short spur off the campground road on the left as you enter the campground. A1 is a bit more shaded by a dense grove of conifers. Several large chunks of granite form a wall at the back of the site. Site A2 is a bit more open and sunlit. Both are great sites, though, especially if you manage to get them both with a larger group or family.

As you move farther along the campground road, site A3 is small but secluded on the sides. It's right across the campground road from the host site. Site A4 is a bit small but surrounded by a dense wall of forest. Site A5 is larger and has a more open feeling. It's open to the road and to the sky. Also, the bathroom and shower building is right behind the site. Site A6 is very open to the campground road and the bathroom buildings.

> *The spectacular new Gilson Pond Campground is yet another reason to visit Monadnock State Park.*

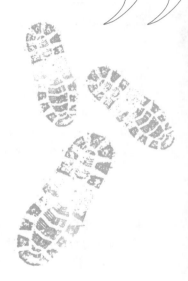

RATINGS

Beauty: ☆☆☆☆☆
Privacy: ☆☆☆☆
Spaciousness: ☆☆☆☆
Quiet: ☆☆☆☆☆
Security: ☆☆☆☆
Cleanliness: ☆☆☆☆☆

ADDRESS: 585 Dublin Rd.
Jaffrey, NH 03452

OPERATED BY: New Hampshire
Division of Parks
and Recreation

INFORMATION: Monadnock State
Park, 603-532-8862

OPEN: Memorial Day–
Columbus Day
(year-round camp-
ing at Monadnock
State Park)

SITES: 35 sites, 5 remote
hike-in sites

EACH SITE: Fire ring with
grate, picnic table;
some sites have
tent platforms

ASSIGNMENT: First-come, first-
served or by res-
ervation: 877-647-
2757 or reserve
america.com

REGISTRATION: At ranger station at
entrance to park

FACILITIES: Flush toilets, coin-
operated showers,
outhouses, water
spigots

PARKING: At sites or smaller
parking areas

FEE: $18–$30

RESTRICTIONS: *Pets:* Not allowed
Fires: Fire rings
only
Alcohol: At sites only
Vehicles: 1 per site
Other: Quiet hours
10 p.m.–7 a.m.;
check out by
11 a.m.; no outside
firewood

After the first few A sites, the campground road separates into the A and B loops, right near the bathroom
and shower building. The campground road is made of
hard-packed gravel and takes quite a turn uphill at the
B loop.

Site B1 is a good-sized site. It's nicely secluded and
has two tent platforms, as do most of the sites set up on
the hilly B area. This ensures you of a solid, flat, dry
place for your tent. Sites B2 and B3 are set well off the
campground road, so they're nicely secluded—especially
site B3. It takes about a 50-foot hike into the site, through
the woods past site B2. Sites B4 and B5 are smaller sites
set closer to the road and fairly close to each other. This
would be a good pair of sites for a larger group.

As you start up the B loop hill, site B6 is set up off
the road at an angle. It's good-sized and fairly secluded.
Sites B7 and B8, set well off the road like sites B2 and B3,
share a deep-woods sense of seclusion, as well as a parking area. Site B9 also has two tent platforms, although
it's a bit smaller and closer to the road than B6. Site B11
is smaller but set well off the road, so it offers a decent
sense of seclusion.

At the bottom of the hill that's part of the B loop
road, site B10 is moderately sized, with a nice sense of
seclusion. Just across the road from B10 is the small
parking area for the five remote hike-in sites.

Moving up the hill, you'll come to site B12, on the
outside of the campground loop. It's dark and shady, set
in a dense grove of conifers. It's beautifully secluded on
all sides and has a nice cool, shady feel. This has to be
one of the best sites here at Gilson Pond.

On the inside of the loop, site B13 is a bit more open
to the road but very well secluded on the sides. It's a
decent-size site, with large granite blocks defining the tent
and picnic table area. B14 is another fairly large and well-
secluded site. It's quite shaded, but a bit of sunlight sneaks
down into the site. Site B15 has a similar arrangement,
although it's a bit smaller than B14.

At the top of a hill amid a grove of white pines, site
B16 has a magnificent layout reminiscent of a Japanese
Zen garden. Two tent platforms are interspersed among
the trees. It's nicely shaded yet open to the sky a bit.
Overall, it's beautiful and very aesthetically arranged.

MAP

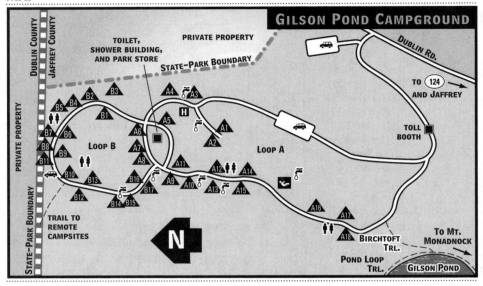

GILSON POND CAMPGROUND

Another fine site near the top of the hill is site B17, set well off the road. It's good-sized, open to the sky yet secluded on the sides. It has its own natural granite "table" as you enter the site.

A short spur in the campground road hosts sites A6 through A8, which face the bathroom and shower building. These three sites are moderately sized and fairly well secluded on the sides, but they are open in front to the road and the bathroom.

As you head toward the top of the hill on the campground road, site A9 is a smaller site but very open to the sky. Site A11 has two tent platforms, but it's quite close to the bathroom as well on the opposite side of the road from sites A6 through A8.

Another beautifully scenic and secluded site is site A10, set down off the road and encircled by dense forest. Site A12 is a smaller, fairly open site. It opens in the back to a small culvert and a rock wall, perfect for scrambling up and around. This natural playground is a nice complement to the man-made one nearby.

It may be small and fairly open to the road, but site A13 has a nice sense of seclusion, especially at the back

GETTING THERE

From NH 124 going north through Jaffrey, turn right on Dublin Road. Follow this 2 miles past the main entrance to Monadnock State Park, to the entrance for Gilson Pond Campground.

GPS COORDINATES

N42° 51.574502'
W72° 3.725817'

of the site. Site A15 is also small yet nicely secluded. It's set off the road in a dense wall of conifers. It's close to the playground, but you can barely see it through the trees. Across the road from site A15 is a mellow, grassy hillside. This is an absolutely perfect spot for stargazing at night. You could just lie back and spend hours watching the sky.

Just below and to the left of this hillside is site A14. The playground is next to the hill, so this would be a perfect site if you have small kids running around and you need to keep an eye on them. A teepee set up at the top of the hill will thrill the kids (of all ages).

A dense wall of mixed coniferous and deciduous forest defines the perimeter of site A16 for a fantastic sense of isolation. It's a bit smaller but beautifully secluded, as it's practically off on its own on the campground loop road.

As you move toward the end of the campground road, you'll find sites A17 and A19. Site A17 is small yet nicely scenic. Its two tent platforms are arranged at different levels and landscaped with large granite blocks. Site A19, the last one on the road, is a good-sized site set back off the road at an angle. The woods are fairly dense here as well, yet you can catch glimpses of Gilson Pond through the trees.

Besides the secluded and scenic nature of the campsites here, the best thing about Gilson Pond is that you can start your hike right from your site—whether you want to take a short hike around the pond or a longer hike up to the summit of Mount Monadnock.

IF YOU START TRAVELING ALONG New Hampshire's fabled Kancamagus Highway heading east or from the Lincoln side to the Conway side, Hancock Campground is the first of the six Kancamagus campgrounds you'll encounter.

It's the only campground along the Kancamagus—or "The Kanc," as the locals call it—that's open year-round. If you come to The Kanc for cross-country skiing or snowshoeing, or if you come to ski at nearby Loon Mountain and you want to do it on the cheap and with a dash of added adventure, pitching your tent at Hancock is the way to go.

Sites 1 through 21 are Hancock's tent-only sites. Within this tent zone, the sites that seem the most off on their own are 10, 12, 14, and 15. Check out these sites first to see if they're available and if they fulfill your need for solitude.

A central parking area is situated near the two loosely spaced loops along which all the tent sites are located. You don't park right at the site in many campgrounds, so be prepared to lug in your gear a short distance. Several areas within the Kancamagus campgrounds have these types of sites, which are perfect for tent camping.

The tent-only sites at Hancock are moderate in size and reasonably spaced. This area also has its own restroom, right across from the sites, in the parking area, so you don't have far to walk when nature calls in the middle of the night.

The rest of the campground's 56 sites are a respectable distance from the tent-only area. You shouldn't discount these sites (22 through 56), even though you might find an RV or two. The sites are fairly spacious, and because the forest is pretty dense here, they're nicely buffered from each other, especially those on the outer end of the loop (sites 35 through 40).

> *Hancock is open year-round for winter camping, and it's close to Lincoln—so it's a good spot for camping with kids.*

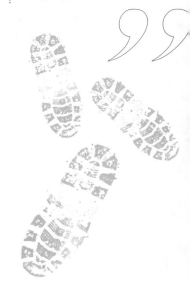

RATINGS

Beauty: ☆ ☆ ☆ ☆
Privacy: ☆ ☆ ☆
Spaciousness: ☆ ☆ ☆
Quiet: ☆ ☆ ☆ ☆
Security: ☆ ☆ ☆ ☆ ☆
Cleanliness: ☆ ☆ ☆ ☆

ADDRESS:	Kancamagus Hwy. Lincoln, NH 03251
OPERATED BY:	U.S. Forest Service, Pro Sport, Inc.
INFORMATION:	Saco Ranger Station, 33 Kancamagus Hwy. (RFD 1, Box 94), Conway, NH 03818; 603-447-5448, icampnh.com
OPEN:	Year-round
SITES:	56
EACH SITE:	Fire ring, picnic table
ASSIGNMENT:	First-come, first-served
REGISTRATION:	Select site, then pay at self-service fee station
FACILITIES:	Flush and vault toilets
PARKING:	At sites or within the parking area for tent sites
FEE:	$22 for 1 vehicle, $5 for extra vehicle
RESTRICTIONS:	*Pets:* Dogs on leash only *Fires:* In fire rings only *Alcohol:* At sites only *Vehicles:* Maximum 2 per site *Other:* Maximum 8 people per site; 14-day maximum stay

These sites are also set within a beautiful birch grove. The first time I visited Hancock Campground was on a classic New England fall day. There wasn't a cloud in the sky, and the air was cool and dry. The sky took on a crystalline azure color. With the combination of the brilliance of the sun and the reflection of the light off the green and yellow leaves of the birch trees, the forest seemed to sparkle.

Also within this loop is where you'll find the trailhead for the short path to the East Branch of the Pemigewasset River, which is a perfect spot to drop a hook in the water (the trail departs between sites 43 and 45 on the outer side of the loop). There are also a few spots where you can drop yourself in the water, but be careful: even late in the summer, that water can be mighty chilly. When you're locating the path, just look beyond the trees for the looming presence of Black Mountain to the south of the campground, and you'll know you're heading in the right direction.

All of the Kancamagus campgrounds are a stone's throw from a pristine river or any number of fabulous hiking trails. It would take you most of the summer to hike them all. Hancock is certainly no different. Right across the street, a trail takes you up and over Potash Knob and Big Coolidge Mountain (and all the way to Mount Flume and Mount Liberty, if you want to go). For a mellower hike, you can walk along the course of the Pemigewasset River.

Hancock is also the campground on the Kancamagus that's closest to civilization. At 5 miles east of Lincoln, it's close enough that you can run over and pick up bread, milk, batteries, or anything else you may have forgotten or run out of. You could also have dinner or see a movie if you've been sleeping in a tent for several nights on end and need a little diversion.

The proximity to Lincoln makes Hancock one of the better Kancamagus campgrounds for families with small children. Kids love camping, but sometimes their tastes for dinner might include a pizza or a burger, and if the weather hasn't been cooperative, an afternoon matinee can be just the antidote for a case of crankiness.

MAP

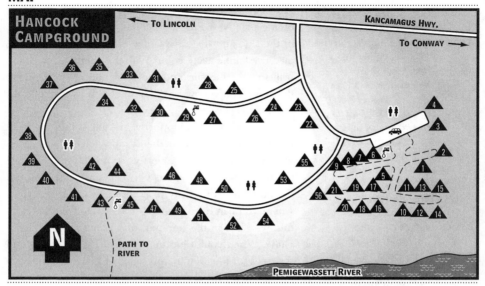

HANCOCK CAMPGROUND

To Lincoln ←

KANCAMAGUS HWY.

To Conway →

PATH TO RIVER

PEMIGEWASSETT RIVER

GETTING THERE

From Lincoln, follow Kancamagus Highway to Hancock Campground, on your right. It's the first campground you'll come to. From Conway, follow Kancamagus Highway to Hancock Campground on your left. From this side, it will be the last campground you come to.

GPS COORDINATES

N44° 3.911755'
W71° 35.689774'

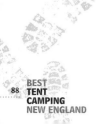

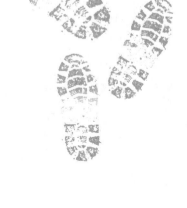

> *Jigger Johnson is the biggest campground on the Kancamagus, but it still has a cozy feel.*

JIGGER **J**OHNSON **IS THE LARGEST** campground on the Kancamagus, but with its well-spaced loops, it affords plenty of room for some high-quality tent camping beneath the statuesque conifers. There's one tent-only loop, which has nine sites reserved for our nylon-bound brethren, but the rest of the campground has plenty of sites where you can experience woodland solitude.

The tent loop is the first one on the left, containing sites 1 through 9—spacious and set amid the forest's rolling contours. This loop also has its own water spigot and restroom, so you won't have to go far for those essentials. Sites 6, 7, and 8, at the far end of the loop, are the most spread out within the tent-only area. Whether you're occupying only one site or have come with several sites' worth of campers, head to the end of the loop first to see what's available.

If the tent loop is full, don't despair: there are plenty of other great sites throughout Jigger Johnson. Most of those along the northeastern end of the campground near the banks of the Swift River are spacious and set within a fairly dense forest. I especially like sites 47, 48, 50, 51, 53, 54, and 57. These feel the most insulated, plus they're close to the water spigots and the Swift River.

The sites on the loop to the right as you enter the campground, while a bit more out in the open, are also excellent spots. True, you run the risk of an RV lumbering up next to you, but if there are already a number of tents in the area and on either side, which is often the case, you know you'll be in for a nice night. Most of the RVs seem to gravitate toward the sites on the main road heading through the campground.

Over on the right-side loop, the shorter trees and lower brush are somewhat sparse. This does open up the whole area at the ground level, but that effect combines with the towering pines that form the tall forest canopy to imbue the forest with a surreal, almost mystical quality.

RATINGS

Beauty: ☆ ☆ ☆ ☆
Privacy: ☆ ☆ ☆
Spaciousness: ☆ ☆ ☆ ☆
Quiet: ☆ ☆ ☆ ☆
Security: ☆ ☆ ☆ ☆
Cleanliness: ☆ ☆ ☆ ☆

This is particularly noticeable as dusk draws near. The sky overhead is still light, and the smoke from the campfires wafts through the trees and up to the forest canopy as darkness sneaks in beneath the pines. A cathedral-like atmosphere pervades this part of the campground in the quiet hours after dinner. The stillness is broken only by the occasional crack of a campfire.

Jigger Johnson, like the other campgrounds along the Kancamagus, is a self-serve kind of place. Enter the campground and find your perfect spot, then return to that odd-looking green cylinder—the "Iron Ranger," in Forest Service vernacular. Here's where you fill in your registration envelope, pay your fee, and slip it through the Iron Ranger's drop slot. If you need to speak with a real person or buy some firewood, you'll find the rangers down the road that leads off to the right just past the Iron Ranger.

This is also where you'll find the showers. Jigger Johnson is the only campground along The Kanc that has coin-operated hot showers, so don't be surprised to find a few people waiting to clean up. There's even a little parking loop (off to the left as you enter the campground) for shower-seekers from the other Kanc campgrounds.

On Saturday evenings throughout the summer, a series of interpretive programs focuses on particular aspects of the local flora and fauna. These can be quite informative and entertaining—the rangers who present the programs truly know their stuff, and they love to share their knowledge. The presentations are usually held in the small, open area off to the left as you're heading down the short road to the showers.

Jigger Johnson is near the intersection of Bear Notch Road and The Kanc, so you could get here easily from Bartlett or from either side of The Kanc. If you run out of something, it's 9 miles to Bartlett and 13 miles to Conway.

The campground is also very close to some classic White Mountain hiking. Turn left out of the campground to get to trailheads for the Champney Falls Trail (which leads to the Three Sisters and the Middle Sister trails) or the Bolles Trail. Turn right on The Kanc out of Jigger Johnson to get to the Oliverian Brook, Downes Brook, Sabbaday Brook, or Sawyer Pond trails. Pack a

KEY INFORMATION

ADDRESS:	33 Kancamagus Hwy. Albany, NH 03818
OPERATED BY:	U.S. Forest Service, Pro Sport, Inc.
INFORMATION:	Saco Ranger Station, 33 Kancamagus Hwy. (RFD 1, Box 94), Conway, NH 03818; 603-447-5448, icampnh.com
OPEN:	Mid May–mid-Oct.
SITES:	73
EACH SITE:	Fire ring, picnic table
ASSIGNMENT:	First-come, first-served
REGISTRATION:	Select site, then pay at self-service fee station
FACILITIES:	Pay showers, flush toilets, water spigots
PARKING:	At sites
FEE:	$22 for 1 vehicle, $5 for extra vehicle
RESTRICTIONS:	*Pets:* Dogs on leash only *Fires:* In fire rings only *Alcohol:* At sites only *Vehicles:* Maximum 2 per site *Other:* Maximum 8 people per site; 14-day maximum stay

MAP

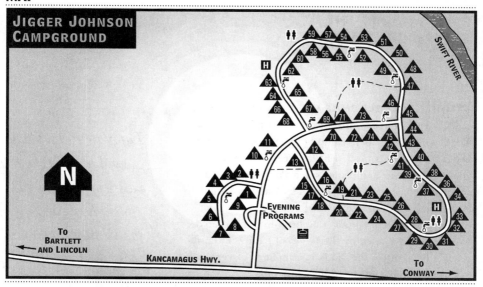

JIGGER JOHNSON CAMPGROUND

N

To
BARTLETT
AND LINCOLN

KANCAMAGUS HWY.

To
CONWAY

SWIFT RIVER

EVENING PROGRAMS

GETTING THERE

From Lincoln, follow Kancamagus Highway to Jigger Johnson Campground, on your left. From Conway, follow Kancamagus Highway to Jigger Johnson Campground, on your right shortly after Bear Notch Road, also on the right.

GPS COORDINATES

N43° 59.502461'
W71° 19.436853'

few extra energy bars and plenty of water if you embark on a hike up the Champney Falls or Middle Sister trails. These lead to Mount Chocorua and the Three Sisters, a beautiful but intense hike.

You can enjoy some great hikes leaving right out of the campground as well—no driving required! The trail that leads down to the banks of the Swift River intersects a trail that runs along the backside of the campground. This mellow path follows the Swift both upstream and downstream for a distance, passing some beautiful bends in the river and through delightfully aromatic groves of birch and pine. It's a great hike to take with kids, because it's relatively flat and there are all sorts of wonderful things to see and experience. Kids can spend hours poking around the banks of the Swift River, and despite its name, this segment of the river is usually fairly tame.

SIMPLY BY VIRTUE OF ITS LOCATION, Lafayette Place Campground is worth including in this guidebook. The fact that it's a superb campground makes it that much better. Lafayette is nestled in the Franconia Valley. As you drive up the Franconia Notch Parkway toward the campground, your view is framed by Cannon Mountain to the left and Mount Lafayette to the right.

Franconia Notch is a veritable sculpture garden displaying works shaped by the forces of nature. From the glaciers that carved the landscape millions of years ago to the tenacious and incessant wind and water, the lay of the land here is as dramatic as anywhere else in New Hampshire. From the waterfalls of the Flume Gorge and the swirling pools of the Basin to Mount Lafayette and the rest of the Presidential range, you could spend weeks here before retracing your steps.

The notch is also headquarters for just about every outdoor activity. There's fly-fishing at nearby Echo Lake (for information on fishing licenses, see Appendix C, page 232); a bike path that winds along the base of the notch; and some fantastic treks for hikers of any ability. Right from the campground, the Lonesome Lake Trail takes you 1,000 feet above the floor of the notch to Lonesome Lake. The trailhead for the 1.5-mile hike is near the entrance to the campground.

There's also a trailhead between sites 67 and 68 that leads to the Basin. From the Basin, you could hike up to Kinsman Falls on Cascade Brook. Follow the 0.5-mile Basin Cascades Trail from the Basin to reach this beautiful and secluded spot.

Lafayette Campground is set beneath a fairly dense forest of conifers and hardwoods. Most of the sites are available by reservation. In fact, the only nonreservable sites are 31 and 93 through 98.

The sites numbered in the upper 40s are very spacious. The forest overhead is open to the sky, which lets

> *Lafayette Place Campground is tucked into the valley of Franconia Notch, home to some of the White Mountains' most spectacular hiking and mountain vistas.*

RATINGS

Beauty: ☆ ☆ ☆ ☆
Privacy: ☆ ☆ ☆
Spaciousness: ☆ ☆ ☆ ☆ ☆
Quiet: ☆ ☆ ☆
Security: ☆ ☆ ☆
Cleanliness: ☆ ☆ ☆ ☆

KEY INFORMATION

a lot of sunlight filter down to the floor of the campsites. Sites 47 and 49 are *too* open, situated as they are right along the campground road. Site 50 is likewise open and right on the road, but it also has the Pemigewasset River running along behind it. Site 51, across the campground road from 50, is also very exposed to the road.

Farther down the campground road on the same side as site 50, site 52 is set off the road and also has the Pemigewasset running behind it. The platform where you'd set up your tent and a picnic table are a bit lower than the road, which adds a degree of seclusion.

The Lonesome Lake Trail runs between sites 53 and 54. Sites 54, 56, and 57 are open to one another and to the neighboring sites. Sites 56 and 58 would be good pair of sites for a larger group needing two contiguous sites. There is a bit of road noise in the background in this part of the campground from the Franconia Notch Parkway. Thankfully, it decreases as you get farther from the road and deeper into the woods.

Sites 61 and 63 are secluded from one another and the neighboring sites. These two sites are also quite spacious. Sites 64 and 66 are another pair of sites that would be well suited for a large group. They are right along the banks of the Pemigewasset, which defines the eastern border of the campground.

Both the ground cover and the forest canopy are less dense in this corner of the campground, so sites 58 through 70 are spacious and sunlit. Lots of breeze flows through here.

A huge maple tree grows up through the center of site 88. This spacious site is on the outside of the campground loop. It's fairly well isolated from the sites on either side, but it is a bit open to the road.

Set off the campground road on a small rise and surrounded by a fairly dense grove of young deciduous trees, site 97 is nicely secluded. However, it's right across the road from the restrooms. Sites 92 and 94 are too open, and 94 is also next to the restroom building on the same side of the road. The Lonesome Lake Trail runs through the campground between sites 93 and 95 on one side of the road and sites 92 and 94 on the other, so these would be good sites to choose if you wanted to be right on the trail, but expect passersby.

MAP

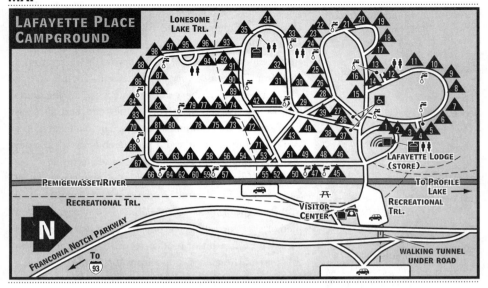

LAFAYETTE PLACE CAMPGROUND

LONESOME LAKE TRL.

PEMIGEWASSET RIVER

RECREATIONAL TRL.

FRANCONIA NOTCH PARKWAY

N

To 93

VISITOR CENTER

LAFAYETTE LODGE (STORE)

TO PROFILE LAKE →

RECREATIONAL TRL.

WALKING TUNNEL UNDER ROAD

The area with sites 73 through 78 is pleasant. These sites feel a bit more privately than some of the sites on the outside of the campground loop. Site 73 is very spacious, open, and sunny. Site 76 is a bit more shaded. Site 75 is also bright, airy, and framed by a wall of maple trees. Alas, site 79 is too close to the restrooms.

Perched at an odd little intersection of the campground loop roads, site 43 has lots of woods surrounding it, with no neighbors on either side. Sites 40 and 29 are also at odd angles in this three-way intersection, but consequently they offer decent privacy. Site 29 is very open and sunny, with large granite boulders framing the back border of the site.

Sites 36 and 37 are set up for wheelchair access. These large sites are set within a grove of fairly dense, mixed forest. Site 27 is very spacious, but it's a bit too open and is on the campground loop road.

Set in the woods around a small grassy field, sites 22 through 26 are open and pastoral. They are not quite as private as the more densely wooded sites, but they're scenic nonetheless. It almost feels as if they were an afterthought.

GETTING THERE

Follow I-93 north to Franconia Notch Parkway. This is a divided highway, so you'll actually drive past the campground and take the next exit off the parkway, then head south. From there, follow the signs for the campground on the right as you head south.

GPS COORDINATES

N44° 8.529754'
W71° 40.976593'

Site 17 is open but secluded and set on a small rise overlooking the field through a loosely spaced grove of young deciduous trees. Sites 15 and 16 are group sites. Right on the grassy field, they offer wide-open prairie camping. They don't offer privacy, but you'd have plenty of room for a group, and a clear shot at the sky for stargazing. Sites 18 and 19 are close to the restrooms but tucked into the woods a bit deeper for privacy. Within this group, sites 11 and 12 are also a bit too close to the restrooms.

The small loop with sites 1 through 10 also surrounds a small, grassy field. These areas make great spots for letting kids run around, throw a Frisbee, or otherwise burn off some steam while you relax. Sites 7 through 10 are quite nice—spacious, open, and fairly well isolated from neighbors. Sites 5 and 6 and sites 1 and 3 would make good pairs of sites for larger groups, as they are open to each other. If you didn't know your neighbors before setting up camp here, you would shortly thereafter.

A small amphitheater and rows of benches are positioned at the entrance to the 1-through-10 loop, where the rangers run nature programs. Check with them as you register to find out what's on the schedule.

THE SITES WITHIN PASSACONAWAY Campground are all quite spacious. This can be both a blessing and a curse. Of all the campgrounds along the Kancamagus, Passaconaway is probably the most conducive to RVs. They are neither catered to (no hookups) nor excluded, but many of the smaller campsites at the other Kancamagus campgrounds naturally keep out the land yachts just by virtue of their size or shape.

On the other hand, the spaciousness of the Passaconaway sites makes them well suited to larger groups or families who need a little extra breathing room. The relatively central location along Kancamagus Highway also puts you in a good spot if you're not sure what part of The Kanc you want to explore. You'll be close to Rocky Gorge, Sabbaday Falls, the Swift River picnic area, and the myriad trailheads spread along the length of this superlative stretch of road.

The forest separating the individual sites at Passaconaway is fairly dense, so even if an RV or a larger group plunks down next to you, you won't see all that much of them. There is lots of undergrowth, which provides seclusion and adds to the silence of the woods. Besides spacious sites, quiet is a prevailing attribute of Passaconaway. All you'll hear are the occasional vehicle zipping past on The Kanc and the soft rush of the wind in the evergreens, punctuated by the chatter of the forest birds and animals.

There are two loops. Sites 1 through 11 are in the loop off to the right as you enter the campground; sites 12 through 33 are in the loop off to the left. The campsites are carved out of a dense forest of mostly coniferous trees, so there's a cool, dark, shaded feeling to the campground.

At the beginning of the 1-to-11 loop, sites 2, 3, and 11 are too open and close to the restrooms for my taste. Sites 5 to 10 are along the outer edge of the loop, off to

> *Passaconaway is a relatively small campground with very spacious sites carved out of a dense evergreen forest.*

RATINGS

Beauty: ✫ ✫ ✫ ✫
Privacy: ✫ ✫ ✫ ✫
Spaciousness: ✫ ✫ ✫ ✫
Quiet: ✫ ✫ ✫ ✫ ✫
Security: ✫ ✫ ✫ ✫
Cleanliness: ✫ ✫ ✫ ✫

KEY INFORMATION

ADDRESS: Kancamagus Hwy. Bartlett, NH 03812

OPERATED BY: U.S. Forest Service, Pro Sport, Inc.

INFORMATION: Saco Ranger Station, 33 Kancamagus Hwy. (RFD 1, Box 94), Conway, NH 03818; 603-447-5448, icampnh.com

OPEN: Mid-May–mid-Oct.

SITES: 32

EACH SITE: Fire ring, picnic table

ASSIGNMENT: First-come, first-served

REGISTRATION: Select site then pay at self-service fee station

FACILITIES: Vault toilets, hand pumps for water

PARKING: At sites

FEE: $20 for 1 vehicle, $5 for extra vehicle

RESTRICTIONS: *Pets:* Dogs on leash only
Fires: In fire rings only
Alcohol: At campsites only
Vehicles: Maximum 2 per site
Other: Maximum 8 people per site, 14-day maximum stay

the right. These sites, mostly by virtue of their location on the outside of the loop road, provide the most solitude. There's simply more room between the sites.

My favorite site on this loop, and one of the best in the campground, is site 10. It's well off on its own, with plenty of space between the neighboring sites on either side. It's also farther off the campground loop road, for an enhanced sense of isolation.

In the 12-to-33 loop, the forest is even denser than in the 1-to-11 loop. On this side of the campground, the forest is composed primarily of pines and maples, many towering to around 80 feet. A moderately dense understory fills in the forest picture and adds to the sense of seclusion between the individual campsites. In this loop, sites 13, 14, and 15 are close to the restroom.

The sites on this loop lie along both the inside and outside of the campground road. A small picnic area sits near site 13. There are pros and cons to this—it's a nice place to have the kids running around close to the campsite, but it could also be a bit noisier during the day. Like most of life's major decisions, whether or not you choose this site will probably be dictated by the presence of little ones.

There's a trailhead right next to site 18. From the Passaconaway Campground, you are near several hiking trails suitable for all ability levels: the long, but not too steep, Sawyer Pond Trail and the shorter but steeper Downes Brook, Sabbaday Brook, and Oliverian Brook trails across The Kanc.

The campground host is at site 19. This is a good place to stop if you need a suggestion for daytime activities, or just to catch a bit of local lore.

The sites numbered in the lower 20s are generally a bit smaller than the rest of Passaconaway's sites and are packed in more tightly. In this group, you're closer to your neighbors and you sacrifice a modicum of privacy and quiet, but you're also less likely to have an RV drop anchor nearby. Still, there is a decent amount of forest buffering these sites.

Huge maples frame sites 22 and 23. Massive maples also grow up within the campsites themselves. You feel as if you're camping among magnificent trees, and you truly are.

MAP

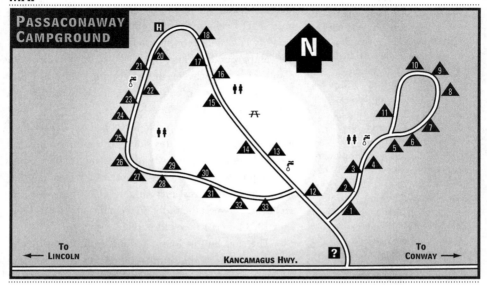

PASSACONAWAY CAMPGROUND

To LINCOLN ←

KANCAMAGUS HWY.

To CONWAY →

GETTING THERE

Site 24 requires a short hike in from where you park. This is the key site here at Passaconaway. The distance from the campground loop road lends it a deep sense of seclusion.

Considering Passaconaway's central location on The Kanc, it's a fine spot to set up camp, especially if you can secure site 10 or site 24.

Passaconaway Campground is almost in the center of Kancamagus Highway. From Lincoln, follow Kancamagus Highway 16 miles to Passaconaway Campground, on the left. From Conway, follow Kancamagus Highway 15 miles to Passaconaway Campground, on the right.

GPS COORDINATES

N43° 59.767227'
W71° 22.163315'

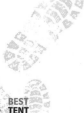

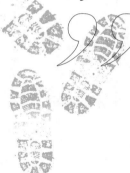

The campground at Pawtuckaway State Park has a lot of sites, but they're split into three different areas, so it has a more intimate feel than you might expect. There are also many sites right on the shores of Pawtuckaway Lake.

RATINGS

Beauty: ☆ ☆ ☆ ☆
Privacy: ☆ ☆ ☆ ☆
Spaciousness: ☆ ☆ ☆ ☆
Quiet: ☆ ☆ ☆
Security: ☆ ☆ ☆ ☆
Cleanliness: ☆ ☆ ☆ ☆

THERE ARE CAMPSITES AT Pawtuckaway State Park that give you the atmosphere of island camping with the ease of car camping. It's a big place, with 191 sites, but the three separate camping areas feel like individual campgrounds.

Horse Island has many of the best sites within the campground—that is to say, the most sites right on the shores of Pawtuckaway Lake. Big Island has some pristine water-view sites, but most of the sites in this area are inland. Neals Cove is near the store, the beach, and the group camping area. These sites, because of their proximity to the beach and playground, are great for families with kids.

Horse Island is home to sites 1 through 80. The island is covered in a fairly dense forest, which lends a nice woodland feel and sense of privacy to most of these sites. The forest is composed of mixed hardwoods and conifers, although it's a bit heavier on the conifers, which fill in the forest and provide cool, dark stillness and seclusion. The sites themselves are clean and spacious, and most have a firm, sandy surface on which to pitch your tent.

I was camped on Horse Island once and had just finished cleaning up from breakfast when a gray heron walked right through my site as if he owned the place. He may well have, but I was too flustered and spellbound to ask him. At Pawtuckaway State Park, Horse Island is where you want to be. The sites that aren't right on the water at least have a water view.

The top-notch Horse Island waterfront sites include 38, 42, 43, 44, 45, 46, and 47. Swimming is not permitted from campsites because Pawtuckaway Lake gets a considerable amount of boat traffic, especially on the weekends. But you could easily launch a canoe or kayak right from your site. Swimming is allowed in the beach and boat-launch areas.

While site 48 is situated near an intersection of the campground road, its lakeside setting more than compensates for any traffic that might pass. Sites 74, 75, and 77 also have nice lakeside settings.

Sites 65 through 70 are clustered at one end of Horse Island. These sites have dramatic lakeside settings. Sites 67 through 69 are perched on their own peninsula jutting out from the southeastern end of the island. If your group is large enough to need three sites and you secure these, you will indeed be set.

You'll find a boat launch and lake access right near sites 58, 60, 62, and 63. These are perfect sites if you like to begin or end your day with a blissful paddle on the still waters of the sleepy lake. Sites 53, 54, and 56 are also primo lakeside spots, set within loosely spaced forest right on the shores of Pawtuckaway Lake, which allows for dramatic views, cool breezes, and shafts of sunlight. I have no scientific evidence to support this, but these lakeside sites seem less buggy than the inland sites to me.

Sites 1, 2, and 25 are right off the campground road leading onto Horse Island, but they offer seclusion, being tucked down off the road amid a dense grove of spruce. Sites 4 and 7 are nicely isolated and set down off the campground loop road facing a small cove. They're in a dense spruce grove where the forest floor gently rolls down to the lakeside. The main body of the lake is around the corner, so it's quieter here as you're removed from the primary thoroughfare through Pawtuckaway Lake. The lake can get pretty heavily populated with ski boats, Jet Skis, and other vessels making more noise than the rhythmic splash of a kayak or canoe paddle.

The sites numbered in the teens are set beneath a loose forest and within view of a small cove. The water is often peaceful and quiet here but does get stirred up during the day. Site 21 is on the water and has a perfectly flat area, offering easy access for launching a canoe or kayak. This site is a paddler's dream. Sites 26 and 27 are nicely isolated from both the road and from other sites, but they're close to each other. They would make a nice pair of sites for a larger family or group.

The Big Island (sounds like Hawaii) section of Pawtuckaway State Park is home to sites 81 through 169. A couple of the sites on the left as you enter the Big Island

KEY INFORMATION

ADDRESS: 128 Mountain Rd. Nottingham, NH 03290

OPERATED BY: New Hampshire Division of Parks and Recreation

INFORMATION: 603-895-3031

OPEN: Mid-May–early Oct.

SITES: 191, plus 5 cabins

EACH SITE: Fire ring, picnic table

ASSIGNMENT: First-come, first-served (sites 81–96 are nonreservable) or by reservation: 877-647-2757, nhstateparks.org, or reserve america.com

REGISTRATION: At campground headquarters

FACILITIES: Flush toilets, hot showers, water spigots, boat launch, canoe and paddleboat rentals

PARKING: At sites

FEE: $25–$30, depending on location of site

RESTRICTIONS: *Pets:* On leash only
Fires: In established fire rings only
Alcohol: At sites only
Vehicles: Parking at campsites only, maximum 2 vehicles per site
Other: Reservations require a 2-night minimum stay, check in between 1 p.m. and 8 p.m., check out by noon, quiet hours 10 p.m.–7 a.m.

MAP

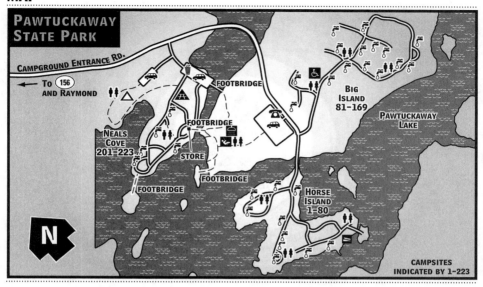

PAWTUCKAWAY STATE PARK

CAMPGROUND ENTRANCE RD.

To 156 AND RAYMOND

FOOTBRIDGE

BIG ISLAND 81-169

PAWTUCKAWAY LAKE

NEALS COVE 201-223

FOOTBRIDGE

STORE

FOOTBRIDGE

FOOTBRIDGE

HORSE ISLAND 1-80

N

CAMPSITES INDICATED BY 1-223

GETTING THERE

Follow NH 101 to NH 156 in Raymond. Follow NH 156 to Mountain Road, and then follow the signs for the park.

GPS COORDINATES

BIG ISLAND
N43° 5.050550'
W71° 9.056854'

NEALS COVE
N43° 5.408127'
W71° 9.527793'

area have steep driveways. Overall, Big Island is hillier than the rest of the campground. There are many sites with steep entries up or down from the road. Just keep that in mind as you select a site so you're not surprised. This is especially true of sites 164 through 169.

RVs and trailers are not expressly prohibited from the sites on Horse Island or Big Island, but those steep, twisty, or narrow entries leading into the sites would preclude one of these behemoths plunking down next to you. Some sites are more open than others, but for the most part, access (or lack thereof) is your best friend.

The Big Island sites are also fairly well isolated from each other, especially sites 162 and 163. These two are situated at the end of a short spur off the campground road and are set within a dense forest of mixed hardwoods and evergreens.

Sites 90 through 93 are set within a deep, dark spruce forest. After site 93, the forest population shifts to deciduous trees. As you walk through the campground road past these sites, it can feel like someone just turned on the lights. You move from the dense, dark spruce forest to the more open and brilliant-green deciduous forest.

MAP

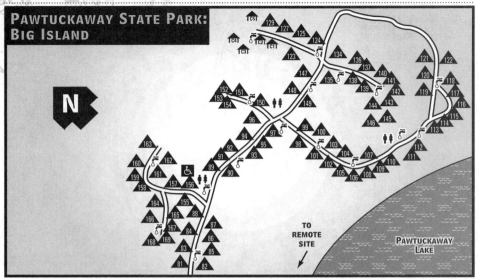

MAP

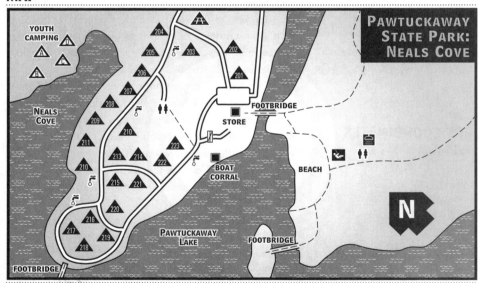

Big Island doesn't have as many water-view sites, but it does have some. Site 108 gets you back on the water. Sites 113 through 118, in their own little loop, all have unimpeded views of the lake and access to launch a canoe or kayak.

The most desirable site within this section is site 122. Feel free to request it, unless, of course, I happen to be traveling to Pawtuckaway that day. Well, in that case you can still request it. We'll just have to share the site—which shouldn't be a problem, since site 122 is absolutely huge.

At the end of the 134-to-146 loop, sites 141 to 143 are quite secluded in their own little cluster. Sites 141 and 142 are actually quite close together but very well situated for a group needing two contiguous sites.

Sites 150 through 152 are up off the road for a solid sense of seclusion. Site 96 lies off an intersection of the road with the one heading to sites 150 to 154, but the site is well isolated by the dense forest and quite large.

Neals Cove is actually the first camping area you come to on the 2-mile access road leading into Pawtuckaway State Park. Most of these sites are smaller but carved out of dense forest, so what they lack in spaciousness they make up for in seclusion. There's a dense, inland feel as you enter this part of the campground, even though you're still quite close to the lake. The beach, camp store, reservation-only group camping areas, picnic area, playground, and baseball field are also near Neals Cove.

Within this part of the campground, sites 206 and up sit along the water within a loosely spaced forest, with dramatic water views and some nice breezes to cool down your campsite. Site 221 is somewhat open to the road but set beneath a dense and statuesque spruce grove. The towering spruce trees populating the forest at Neals Cove give the woods a majestic feel. A footbridge next to site 218 leads onto another small island. This island doesn't have any campsites, but it's a perfect spot to hike out to with lunch or to just sit and watch the lake in the early morning or at dusk.

THE WOODS AND THE WATER are a powerful combination. Pillsbury State Park has both, and in just the right proportions—a series of crystalline ponds cast against a dense blanket of forest like scattered jewels. Although it's part of the New Hampshire state-park system, Pillsbury is a little-known gem. It rests quietly in the deep forest just south of the far more popular and more frequently visited Sunapee State Park, and that's just fine.

When I first entered this campground, I was immediately struck with a moral and ethical dilemma: *Do I really want to tell anyone else about this place?* I honestly didn't ruminate on this for long, though. After considering the proclivities and desires of the sort of reader who would buy this book and would naturally seek out magical spots like this, I had to include Pillsbury State Park. There isn't a bad site in the whole place, and many of the sites are elevated to paradise status, especially those at the water's edge.

As soon as you pull into the lengthy access road, which winds along the shores of Butterfield Pond and then May Pond, you'll know you've found someplace special. If you've come to fully immerse yourself in the solitude of the deep wilderness, you have most definitely come to the right place. The campsites are spread out along this road, either alone or in clusters. Most are right on or very close to the shores of May Pond. Several are inland, tucked into the dense forest that surrounds the ponds and marshy areas in the park.

The first sites you'll come to are 1 and 1A, off the main access road to the left, at the end of a short drive. You can park at site 1, but 1A is a walk-in site. These are the only two sites on the shores of Vickery Pond, one of the smaller ponds in the park. Want to be off by yourself? Bring a small group, even just two couples; you'll have this pond to yourself.

> *Many of Pillsbury State Park's campsites are so spread out that you'll feel as if you have the campground to yourself.*

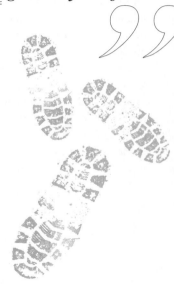

RATINGS

Beauty: ☆ ☆ ☆ ☆ ☆
Privacy: ☆ ☆ ☆ ☆ ☆
Spaciousness: ☆ ☆ ☆ ☆ ☆
Quiet: ☆ ☆ ☆ ☆ ☆
Security: ☆ ☆ ☆ ☆ ☆
Cleanliness: ☆ ☆ ☆ ☆ ☆

ADDRESS: Route 31
Washington, NH
03280

OPERATED BY: New Hampshire
Division of Parks
and Recreation

INFORMATION: 603-863-2860

OPEN: Mid May–late Oct.

SITES: 41 sites, including
2 canoe sites

EACH SITE: Fire ring

ASSIGNMENT: All but 5 sites are
available by reser-
vation only (877-
647-2757, 603-271-
3628, nhstateparks
.org, or reserve
america.com); the
rest are first-come,
first-served

REGISTRATION: At campground
headquarters

FACILITIES: Pit toilet, water
spigots, play-
ground, canoe
rentals

PARKING: At sites or in parking areas for hike-
in or canoe sites

FEE: $16–$23

RESTRICTIONS: *Pets:* Dog on leash
only
Fires: In fire rings
only
Alcohol: At sites only
Vehicles: Parking at
or near campsites,
only 2 vehicles
per site
Other: Reservations
require a 2-night
minimum stay;
check in between
1 p.m. and 8 p.m.,
check out by
noon; quiet hours
10 p.m.–7 a.m.

Next along the main road is site 2. Although this site is right off the access road, it, too, is completely on its own. This is a great spot if you want to enjoy waterfront camping in relative solitude, because it's perched on the shore of Butterfield Pond. The only other site on this pond is site 39, on the other side of the pond—accessible only by canoe or kayak.

Sites 3 through 7 are grouped together in a small cluster farther up the road on the right. These are set on a small peninsula that helps define the border between Butterfield Pond and May Pond. There is also a pair of pit toilets here. Farther along the road, also waterside, is the small loop with sites 9 through 19. These sites are within the largest and most densely packed cluster of sites in the park, but even these are quite nice. Within this loop, go for sites 11, 12, and 14, as they are right on the shores of May Pond. Site 15 is pretty darn close to the pond as well.

Toward the end of the campground road are sites 23, 24, 26, and 40. At site 40, you park across from a footbridge over a small stream. Cross the bridge and turn right on the footpath that leads down to site 40, nestled right on the shoreline of the pond. It's well worth every trip to the car. You'll have your own slice of forest right on your own corner of the pond.

If you're a paddler, do what you can to reserve either site 38 or 39. These are the canoe- and kayak-accessible sites. It's just a short paddle across May Pond to site 38 or Butterfield Pond to site 39. Then you'll feel as if you're camping on an island, and you'll have your vessel right there to explore the interconnected Butterfield and May ponds. Some of the same considerations of island camping apply here, such as the pack-in, pack-out ethic. Be sure you've brought everything you need. A trip back to your vehicle will take some effort.

Besides the paddling, wildlife viewing, and relaxing by the shores of the pond, there is a massive network of hiking trails winding through Pillsbury State Park. This park and its trails form part of the Monadnock–Sunapee Greenway, a 51-mile route that connects the two peaks. It's sort of like a mini (very mini) Appalachian Trail.

The Monadnock–Sunapee Trail is the main trail here. You could get quite far along the trail, so set a

MAP

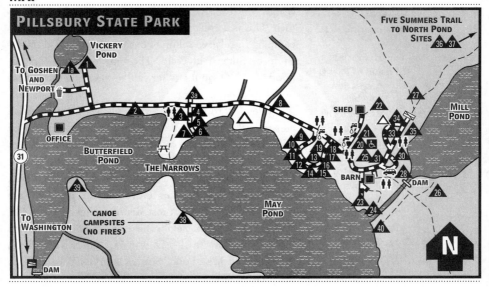

predetermined turnaround time to leave yourself enough light to make it back to camp. The peaks of Kittredge and Lovewell mountains, both within Pillsbury State Park, are good day hikes from the campground on this trail. The Ayers Pond Trail is a nice long route that ultimately leads out to its namesake body of water.

Back at camp, the mirrorlike surface of a pond will reflect the last light of the day. You may be treated to the sight of a great blue heron swooping down for a final landing, or you might spot a moose wandering about the wetlands. Pillsbury State Park is a true wilderness getaway.

GETTING THERE

Follow NH 31 from Hillsborough and Washington. The park is on the right, about 15 miles past the center of Washington.

GPS COORDINATES

N43° 13.883858'
W72° 7.291131'

28
WILDWOOD
CAMPGROUND

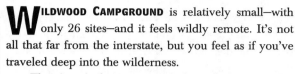

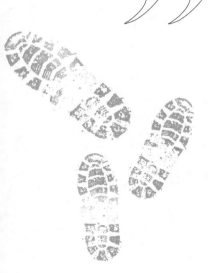

The sense of isolation and remoteness at Wildwood makes this gem well worth the trip.

WILDWOOD **CAMPGROUND** is relatively small—with only 26 sites—and it feels wildly remote. It's not all that far from the interstate, but you feel as if you've traveled deep into the wilderness.

There's a fairly consistent feel to all the sites. The sites are carved out of older forest of mixed conifers and deciduous trees, with lots of white pine, spruce, maple, and beech. The sites are also of moderately consistent size—only a few are larger than the rest.

There are two loops within the campground layout. Most of the sites are somewhat open to the road, but since this is a fairly small and quiet campground, that tends to not matter as much. The sites are mostly secluded on the sides from neighboring sites.

During the day you'll hear some occasional road noise from NH 112, but at night that fades off to nothing. The dense and towering forest infuses the campground with a deep sense of darkness. You'll catch only glimpses of the night sky overhead through gaps in the forest canopy directly over your site.

As you move into the campground, sites 1 and 2 are very open to each other and to the campground road. They're closer to NH 112 than any other sites in the campground as well. These two would make a good pair of sites for a larger group.

Site 3 is at the head of the first loop. It's fairly secluded by the dense forest and fairly well set off on its own. Site 4 is very open and is the first site you'll come to on the right as you move up the right-side loop of the campground road. It has a nice grassy surface on the floor of the site and is framed by several huge white pines. Site 5 is a bit smaller but is nicely secluded by the forest.

Site 6 has a more open feel, and it's also set closer to the campground loop road. Site 7 is similarly open to the road but nicely secluded on the sides. It's also right across from a water spigot, so you might get a bit of foot

RATINGS

Beauty: ☆ ☆ ☆ ☆
Privacy: ☆ ☆ ☆
Spaciousness: ☆ ☆ ☆
Quiet: ☆ ☆ ☆ ☆
Security: ☆ ☆ ☆ ☆
Cleanliness: ☆ ☆ ☆ ☆

traffic coming by your site. Site 8 is very nicely secluded, requiring a short walk into the site from where you park your car. It's shaded on all sides by a ring of large trees and open to the sky above. It's also a bit larger than the surrounding sites.

A dense wall of spruce and pine surrounds site 9. It also has a nice grassy surface on the site floor. It is a bit open to the road, though. Site 10 is a bit smaller but set off from the road. It's punctuated by a small hill at the back of the site. It's also across from the bathroom building. Site 11 is a bit larger than site 10 but also right across from the bathrooms. Sunlight filters down to these sites during the day through the opening in the forest canopy above the sites.

Being set back off the road affords site 12 a nice sense of seclusion. It's also more open to the sky than some of the other sites here. Site 13 is down off the road. It's fairly close to the bathroom but secluded from the road. The site has a separate driveway and a short path leading to it. The host site is 14.

Site 15 is huge and framed by pines and maples, but it feels quite open to the road. Site 16 sits where the campground loop roads rejoin. It's a smaller site but fairly well secluded from the road and from site 17. Site 17 is quite large, although it is fairly open to the road where the campground roads rejoin at a small intersection. Site 18 is of moderate size, with a grassy surface on the site floor. It's also quite open to the sky. Site 19 is smaller but set well off the road so it has a greater sense of seclusion. It also requires about a 50-foot hike in. This is one of the nicer, more secluded sites at Wildwood.

Site 21 has an open feel. It's secluded on the sides but open to the road and the Dumpster across the road. Site 20 is also across the road from site 21. It's near the Dumpster but fairly secluded on the sides. Site 22 is set well back from the road, so it feels quite secluded by the dense forest. It's also set down from the road somewhat, so there's a short walk into the site.

A nice amount of sunlight filters down to site 23. It's a smaller site that's set off the road a bit. Site 24 is a bit larger, but also more open to the road and the bathroom building. Site 25 is a moderately sized site. Site 26 is very open to the road and to site 25 as well.

KEY INFORMATION

ADDRESS:	NH 112 Lincoln, NH 03251
OPERATED BY:	U.S. Forest Service, Pro Sport, Inc.
INFORMATION:	Pemigewassett Ranger Station, 603-745-3816, icampnh.com
OPEN:	Mid-May– Columbus Day
SITES:	26
EACH SITE:	Fire ring with grate, picnic table
ASSIGNMENT:	First-come, first-served
REGISTRATION:	Pay at ranger station at entrance to park
FACILITIES:	Vault toilets, water spigots
PARKING:	At sites or in parking area
FEE:	$16 for 1 vehicle, $5 for extra vehicle
RESTRICTIONS:	*Pets:* On leash or in cage at all times *Fires:* Fire rings only *Alcohol:* At sites only *Vehicles:* 1 per site, $5 for extra vehicle *Other:* Quiet hours 10 p.m.–7 a.m.; check out by 10 a.m.

MAP

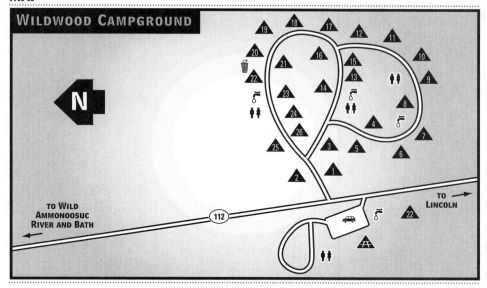

WILDWOOD CAMPGROUND

GETTING THERE

Follow I-93 north to Exit 32, NH 112 (Kancamagus Highway), in Lincoln. Head west on NH 112 for 9 miles past the town of North Woodstock, passing Lost River on your right. The campground will be on the same side of the road, 4 miles past Lost River.

GPS COORDINATES

N44° 4.549999'
W71° 47.599983'

As at many other White Mountain National Forest campgrounds, you register and pay at the "Iron Ranger" as you enter the campground. After you've found your site, grab an envelope at the self-serve kiosk and slip your payment into the green iron container.

Several trailheads lead right off NH 112 as you're heading to Wildwood Campground from Woodstock. Keep your eyes open or bring along the AMC's White Mountain hiking guide to plan your trips.

While you're here, check out the Lost River—a long series of decks and walkways that lead you through a series of caverns and passages, through massive chunks of granite casually left behind by retreating glaciers. There are fascinating rock formations, partly due to the glaciers and partly due to the incessant carving force of the water rushing through them. It's also probably the coolest place you could be on a steamy summer afternoon.

If that's not cool enough for you, head across NH 122 from the campground and make your way down to the banks of the Wild Ammonoosuc River. The river flow may not always be wild, but it is always wildly cold. If that water doesn't cool you down, you must be part polar bear.

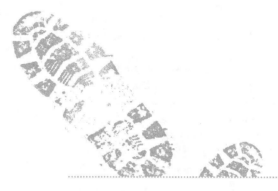

VERMONT

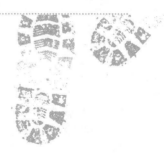

29
BRANBURY
STATE PARK

THERE ARE TWO SEPARATE CAMPING AREAS at Branbury State Park. One is pretty nice, but the other is positively spectacular. Branbury State Park is on the eastern shore of Lake Dunmore, and there's plenty to do on this beautiful central Vermont lake: paddling, fishing, sailing, swimming, or just sitting on a beach chair burrowing your feet into the sand (for information on fishing licenses, see Appendix C, page 232).

The camping area near the lake is set on an open field back from the beach. For the Lake Dunmore side of the campground, the privacy rating is one star, since it's an open field. A few trees are spread out within the field, but for the most part, the only thing between you and the neighboring sites is air. The campsites across the street rate a four on the privacy scale, and some a solid five.

Sites 1 through 17 are the open sites near the lake. These are pleasant, as they're close to the lake and you'll get some cool breezes, but they are all quite similar and all very open. If you prefer seclusion, the campsites across the street (sites 20 through 41 and the lean-to sites) are where you want to be. This portion of the campground is set within a beautiful mixed forest of old and young trees. This loop has some scenic and secluded sites, as well as a few lean-tos. In Vermont State Parks style, the lean-tos are all named for tree varieties: Elm, Spruce, Oak, and so on. These are unobtrusively mixed in with the tent sites.

Site 25 isn't bad. It's slightly elevated from the road, but it's right at the entrance to this side of the campground where campers drive in, so it lacks privacy and quiet. Sites 27 and 28 are probably the least private of the sites on this side, as they have the main road (VT 53) on one side and the campground loop road on the other. Travel just a bit farther up this loop, though, and the sites become increasingly gorgeous.

> *Here you can choose between campsites on a grassy field near the lake or nestled deep in the woods.*

RATINGS

Beauty: ✩ ✩ ✩ ✩
Privacy (west): ✩
Privacy (east): ✩ ✩ ✩ ✩ ✩
Spaciousness: ✩ ✩ ✩ ✩
Quiet: ✩ ✩ ✩ ✩
Security: ✩ ✩ ✩ ✩
Cleanliness: ✩ ✩ ✩ ✩

KEY INFORMATION

ADDRESS: 3570 Lake Dunmore Rd. Salisbury, VT 05733

OPERATED BY: Vermont Agency of Natural Resources–Department of Forests, Parks, and Recreation

INFORMATION: 802-247-5925 (summer), 888-409-7579 (Oct.–May)

OPEN: Memorial Day–Columbus Day

SITES: 36 tent sites, 7 lean-to sites

EACH SITE: Fire ring, picnic table

ASSIGNMENT: First-come, first-served or by reservation: 888-409-7579, vtstateparks.com

REGISTRATION: At ranger station

FACILITIES: Flush toilets, water, coin-operated hot showers, sandy beach on Lake Dunmore, boat rentals

PARKING: At sites

FEE: $16–$20 for tent sites, $23–$27 for lean-tos

RESTRICTIONS: *Pets:* Dogs on leash only
Fires: In fire rings only
Alcohol: At sites only
Vehicles: At sites only
Other: Reservations require 4-night minimum stay; check in after 2 p.m., check out by 11 a.m.; quiet hours 10 p.m.–7 a.m.; maximum 8 people per site

Site 32 is nicely isolated, situated on the inside of the campground loop near the Birch lean-to. Sites 29 and 31 are even farther up on the spectacular scale. These well-isolated sites are on a small rise from the campground road and are surrounded by thick forest. Site 30 sits in the middle of these two sites, so it's more open, but it's still a fine site. Sites 29 and 31 on either side are set far back enough in the woods that you won't be too close to your neighbors.

Farther up the loop are several sites set against small granite cliff walls. Sites 36 and 37 are tucked right against these ledges. The whole side of the loop here is quite dramatic in its scenery, thanks to the cliffs, forest, and gently rolling terrain.

Three sites on this side of the Branbury State Park campground are set at the end of cul-de-sacs within the campground: sites 34, 41, and 21. Site 34 is perfectly situated for deep wilderness isolation. It's nestled in a dense grove of conifers, so it feels like a campsite from some deep mystical woods out of J. R. R. Tolkien's Middle-earth.

Site 41 is also set off on its own in a pine grove up against the cliffs. This site is next to the Spruce lean-to. Sites 39 through 41 are interspersed with the shelters against and among the cliffs. Site 39 is an isolated site, even though it sits right next to the Oak Shelter.

Then we come to site 21 (glorious cinematic music should be playing in your head right now). This couldn't possibly be a more perfect place to spend a few days camping. You'll walk a short distance to lug in your gear. Make sure to drop your stuff and just look around as you walk into the site. You'll feel as if you've entered a cathedral. The site is majestically framed by statuesque spruce trees and set against a steep cliff wall. As if that's not enough, Sucker Brook softly splashes by right behind the site. You'll fall asleep to the sounds of the stream as it runs down from the Falls of Lana toward Lake Dunmore.

When I was chatting with the Vermont Youth Conservation Corps members working in the ranger station in early spring, the coveted site 21 was already reserved for most of the summer. Plan years in advance, do a sun dance, and try to get yourself some time in this excellent site. You'll be glad you did!

MAP

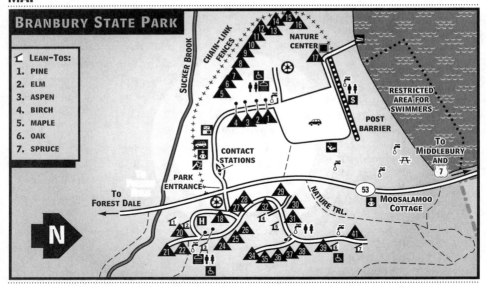

BRANBURY STATE PARK

LEAN-TOS:
1. PINE
2. ELM
3. ASPEN
4. BIRCH
5. MAPLE
6. OAK
7. SPRUCE

SUCKER BROOK

CHAIN-LINK FENCES

NATURE CENTER

RESTRICTED AREA FOR SWIMMERS

POST BARRIER

To MIDDLEBURY AND 7

CONTACT STATIONS

PARK ENTRANCE

To FOREST DALE

N

NATURE TRL.

53

MOOSALAMOO COTTAGE

While most Vermont State Parks have a two-night minimum for reservations, Branbury State Park has a four-night minimum. That should be fine though, especially if you get yourself into site 21. Otherwise, consider sites 20, 22, 29, 31, 34, and 41 for the most secluded wilderness experience. Once you land there, you won't want to leave for at least four nights!

Besides the fishing, paddling, and basking in the sun on the shores of Lake Dunmore, the hiking in and around Branbury State Park is as dramatically beautiful as site 21. A nature trail loops up and over the small cliffs at the back of the wooded side of the campground. There are two hikes in particular that you won't want to miss if you're spending at least a couple of days here: the 1.5-mile, occasionally strenuous hike up to Rattlesnake Point, a rock promontory overlooking the forest and Lake Dunmore; and the relatively easy 1-mile hike up to the Falls of Lana, over which Sucker Brook flows on its way toward site 21 and Lake Dunmore.

GETTING THERE

From Middlebury, travel south on US 7, then south on VT 53 until you see signs for the park.

GPS COORDINATES

N43° 54.333987'
W73° 3.965321'

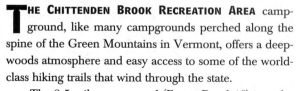

> *This is a spectacularly scenic and isolated campground set deep within the woods of the Green Mountain National Forest.*

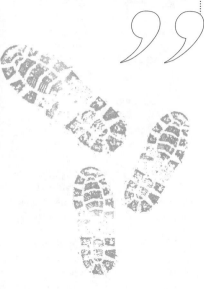

THE **CHITTENDEN BROOK RECREATION AREA** campground, like many campgrounds perched along the spine of the Green Mountains in Vermont, offers a deep-woods atmosphere and easy access to some of the world-class hiking trails that wind through the state.

The 2.5-mile access road (Forest Road 45) into the campground is quite a trip in and of itself. It leads up and over a ridge, with Chittenden Brook running on either side along the way. Farther up, as you near the campground, the road falls off steeply to the right. Even though the forest is dramatically beautiful here, keep your eyes on the road.

Chittenden Brook is one of those campgrounds (and there are certainly plenty in New England) where there isn't a bad site in the place. It's an intimate campground with only 17 sites, which means it can fill up quickly. Once you're there, it's calm and quiet and has a delightful sense of solitude.

The whole campground is situated near the ridgeline of the Green Mountains, the course followed by the nearby Long and Appalachian trails. You are at a moderate elevation in the Green Mountains, so the forest isn't quite as towering here. Consequently, lots of light filters down into the sites. There's also the ever-present rush of Chittenden Brook, punctuated by the staccato chirping of the forest birds. It's a profoundly peaceful combination.

Site 1 is down off the road, near the restrooms but set off on its own enough to be fairly well isolated. Continuing along the campground loop road, sites 2 through 5 are fairly close together, but each has plenty of room. These sites have an open feel, and are probably the least isolated sites in the campground. Still, even these offer a reasonable sense of seclusion.

While it doesn't have a lot of dense forest surrounding it, site 6 is nicely isolated, as it is set off from the other campsites. It's also situated right next to a trailhead

RATINGS

Beauty: ✿ ✿ ✿ ✿ ✿
Privacy: ✿ ✿ ✿ ✿ ✿
Spaciousness: ✿ ✿ ✿ ✿ ✿
Quiet: ✿ ✿ ✿ ✿ ✿
Security: ✿ ✿ ✿ ✿
Cleanliness: ✿ ✿ ✿ ✿

between sites 6 and 7 that leads to the Chittenden Brook Trail, the Beaver Pond Trail, and the Campground Loop Trail. You can hike right out of your campsite. Site 7 is larger, so it would be perfect for a group or large family. It's also next to the restroom.

The tent platform for site 8 is off the campground loop and back in the woods, so this site scores higher on the solitude and isolation scale. Given its location and the trees around the site, you probably won't even be able to see your neighbors. Sites 9 and 10 are right across the campground loop road from each other. Both are pretty, spacious sites surrounded by trees that lend a sense of isolation on either side, although the front of the campsite is open.

Sites 11 and 12 are right next to each other and have a loosely spaced, fairly open forest in between, so these would be good sites if you're with a group large enough to need or want two sites. Sites 13 and 15 are set off from the campground loop road, with a short path leading to the tent platform. These sites not only provide a sense of wilderness and isolation but are also extra-scenic since they are set within groves of young decidu- ous trees, loaded with brilliant green leaves bouncing around in the sunlight.

Sites 16 and 17 are my favorites at Chittenden Brook Recreation Area. In site 16, the tent platform is set off the road, and then from there the space with the picnic table and fire ring is set down farther still, so both your sleeping spot and hanging-out spot are off on their own. There's also a buffer of woods between sites 16 and 17 and on either side. Site 17 is a bit more level but still mar- velously isolated, quite spacious, and surrounded by a cloak of young trees. It's near the end of the campground loop road and close to the recycling station. These recy- cling stations are very much in evidence within the Green Mountain National Forest campgrounds and recreation areas. Bravo to that!

This is the place to make base camp if you're plan- ning on exploring portions of the Long Trail or Appala- chian Trail. Trailheads lead right out of the campground. As you drive in on the access road, you'll pass other trailheads also leading off toward the Long Trail.

ADDRESS:	Forest Road 45 VT 73 Chittenden, VT 05737
OPERATED BY:	Green Mountain National Forest
INFORMATION:	Rochester Ranger District, 99 Ranger Rd., Rochester, VT 05767-9431; 802-767-4261
OPEN:	Memorial Day–Labor Day
SITES:	17
EACH SITE:	Fire ring with grill, picnic table
ASSIGNMENT:	First-come, first-served
REGISTRATION:	Pay at self-serve fee station
FACILITIES:	Pit toilets, no drinking water available
PARKING:	At sites
FEE:	$10
RESTRICTIONS:	*Pets:* On leash only *Fires:* In fire rings only *Alcohol:* At sites only *Vehicles:* Maximum 2 per site; national forest closed to ATVs *Other:* Quiet hours 10 p.m.–6 a.m.; check out by 2 p.m.; 14-day maximum stay; pack out all trash

MAP

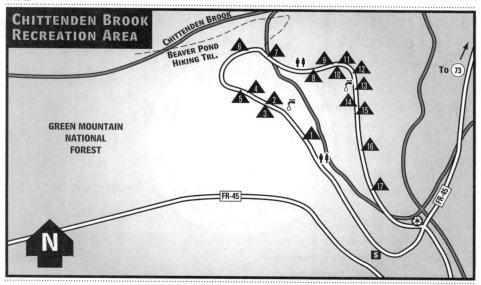

GETTING THERE

Follow VT 73 to Forest Road 45 and the sign for Chittenden Brook Recreation Area, which will be on the left if you're heading west on VT 73, or on the right if you're heading east. Follow FR 45 about 2.5 miles to the campground.

GPS COORDINATES

N43° 49.449213'
W72° 54.564950'

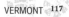

31
COOLIDGE STATE PARK

WHEN YOU'RE HIKING THROUGH the gentle trails of Coolidge State Park (so named for the nearby birthplace of Calvin Coolidge, 30th president of the United States), you'll come across lots of old stone walls and what's left of foundations. Close your eyes for a moment and imagine what this area was like when the homes of farmers stood here. The land upon which you're hiking and camping looked a lot different just 100 years ago. What was once agricultural land has been thoroughly reclaimed by the forest's persistent growth.

The campground at Coolidge State Park is set within a dense, mixed forest of mostly deciduous trees. There's a stately character to the forest, as most of the trees tower 75 to 100 feet overhead. Most of the trees are maple, birch, and pine. The tent sites are generally very spacious, with lots of space and trees between most of the sites, so the sense of seclusion is supreme. The campground is very quiet. The only sounds you'll hear are the woodland birds and the breezes rustling through the trees.

Unlike most other state-park campgrounds in Vermont, this one has two distinct areas for most of the lean-tos and the tent sites. The White Birch, Alder, and Poplar lean-tos are the only three mixed in with the tent sites. The White Birch lean-to is at the head of the tent loop, the Alder across from site 4, and the Poplar off the main campground road.

While it's smaller than the other low-numbered sites, site 1 is well isolated. The main campground road runs behind the site, but you won't notice it once the sun sinks beneath the trees. It's also directly across the campground loop road from site 2, which is framed by a grove of spruce and young deciduous trees. A huge, grand old pine tree guards the entrance to site 2, its hanging branches reminiscent of a weeping willow's.

There's a fairly well-isolated air about site 3, although it's close to site 2. A decent amount of forest separates the

> *The character of the forest and the views of the surrounding hillside make this park a gem.*

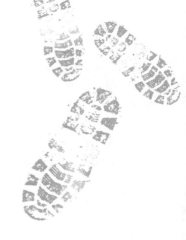

RATINGS

Beauty: ✪ ✪ ✪ ✪
Privacy: ✪ ✪ ✪ ✪ ✪
Spaciousness: ✪ ✪ ✪ ✪
Quiet: ✪ ✪ ✪ ✪ ✪
Security: ✪ ✪ ✪ ✪
Cleanliness: ✪ ✪ ✪ ✪

KEY INFORMATION

two, and both are very spacious. Site 4 is also spacious, and it's right across the road from the Alder lean-to. The site is framed by a grove of young deciduous trees and a few older spruce. Site 5 is another well-isolated one. It's at least 100 feet from sites on either side, but it is open to the back, and you can see the restrooms behind it. Site 6 is just off the campground road. It's also fairly close to the restrooms.

The trailhead for the CCC (Civilian Conservation Corps) Trail is right across from site 7. This is a convenient site for easy access to the hiking trails that wind throughout the park, but expect passing foot traffic. Sites 7 and 8 are somewhat close together and up off the campground loop road. Site 9 is very open and has a small, grassy area within. It's right next to site 10, so unlike most of the campground, there isn't much privacy between 9 and 10. These two pairs of sites would suit large groups or families.

Site 11 is another open and spacious spot. Site 12 is smaller and more secluded, surrounded by a dense grove of young deciduous trees. Site 13 is tucked far off the campground road, so it provides a feeling of isolation, even though it's right next to a short footpath that leads up to the restrooms.

Sites 14 and 15 share an entranceway, but there's enough space and forest between the two to afford sufficient privacy. Both sites are spacious and set far off the road. Site 15 offers a fabulous sense of solitude, boasting a grassy area, plus a brook.

There isn't much privacy between sites 16 and 17. However, there's plenty of room on either side of both sites, so they're well isolated from the rest of the campground, if not from each other—another possibility for groups. Site 17 is set off the road a bit and has a grassy surface in its center. Several maples grow up through the site, and it's framed by shorter deciduous trees—mostly maple and birch—and by ferns at the ground level for an added sense of seclusion. The ferns give the site a primeval feel and fill in the forest with their brilliant green leaves. When the sunlight filters down on a clear day, the forest looks as if it's glowing green.

Site 18 is a bit smaller than 17 but also has a grassy surface. Site 19 is spacious, and there's plenty of forest on either side of the site but not too much privacy from the road. I'm always willing to sacrifice a bit of spaciousness for more forest and a deeper sense of seclusion.

Sites 20 through 23 have a similar character. Site 20 is up off the road. This is a moderately spacious site with a grassy surface. Sites 22 and 23 are across the road from each other. Site 23A is a lug-in site up off the road. It's almost a part of Site 23, so if you don't know your neighbors in site 23 before your trip, you will before long. Site 23A isn't huge, but it's set way off from the road and the rest of the campground. It's surrounded by a dense, low wall of ferns and a grove of slender young spruce trees. It has lots of privacy on all sides, save where it abuts site 23.

One of the last sites on this part of the campground loop road is site 24. This is by far the most isolated site within the loop. It's perfectly situated to afford a wilderness experience, as it's surrounded by dense forest and is a good distance from its neighbors. It's not the most spacious site, but it's marvelously well isolated.

Site 25 poses a tradeoff. It sits way off on its own, but it's near the point where the campground loop road rejoins the main state-park road. It's moderately spacious and well isolated from the other sites, but it is right at that intersection.

Between the tent loop and the lean-to loop is a little playground near the ranger station as you enter the park—a good thing to keep in mind if you're camping with little ones. The lean-to loop has very dense forest coverage as well. Most of the lean-tos are quite well isolated from each other, although some are positioned in pairs, like Cherry and Larch, or groups, like Beech, Basswood, and Apple. Between the dense forest and the loose spacing, the individual lean-to sites offer isolation, especially the Sumac, Willow, and Butternut lean-tos. It also bears mentioning that the Cedar lean-to is wheelchair-accessible.

The Ash lean-to has an outrageously scenic view of the opposing hillsides and valley. This alone makes it worth keeping the tent packed, and hopping in one of these lean-tos. The Aspen, Boxelder, Beech, Basswood, Elm, and Hawthorn lean-tos also share this dramatic view. All these lean-tos face out toward the hills, which would be the first thing you'd see in the morning. I couldn't imagine a nicer way to greet the day.

Once you're up and about, whether you've spent the night in your tent or in a lean-to, there's plenty of great hiking right within the park. Try the 0.75-mile CCC Trail, which connects the tent area and the lean-to area for a mellow morning hike. Then try the 1.5-mile trail to the summit of the 2,174-foot Slack Hill and treat yourself to lunch with a commanding view of the surrounding hills.

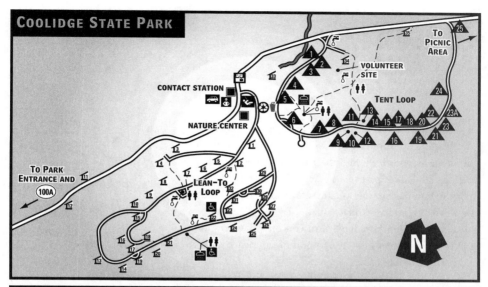

COOLIDGE STATE PARK

LEAN-TOS:

1. SHADBLOW	8. OAK	15. HACKBERRY	22. CEDAR	29. TAMARACK
2. HEMLOCK	9. BALSAM	16. SUMAC	23. DOGWOOD	30. WALNUT
3. CHERRY	10. SYCAMORE	17. BUTTERNUT	24. ELM	31. LOCUST
4. LARCH	11. BLUEBERRY	18. WILLOW	25. BASSWOOD	32. CHESTNUT
5. SPRUCE	12. SAPLING	19. ASPEN	26. BEECH	33. ALDER
6. PINE	13. HORNBEAM	20. BOXELDER	27. APPLE	34. WHITE BIRCH
7. MAPLE	14. ASH	21. HAWTHORN	28. HICKORY	35. POPLAR

GETTING THERE

Follow VT 100 (the skier's highway) to VT 100A in Plymouth. Follow VT 100A about 2 miles to the sign for the park, on the right.

GPS COORDINATES

N43° 33.088911'
W72° 41.836796'

YOU CAN'T HELP BUT NOTICE the steep embankment leading up from one side of the road and down from the other as you drive into the Emerald Lake State Park campground. This place was essentially carved out of the hillside. It makes for a dramatic setting, but consequently, a steep bank encircles many of the camping areas here, so keep an eye on any little ones you may have running around. You'll hear a little road noise from nearby US 7, but hardly any at night.

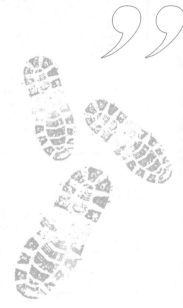

> *Emerald Lake State Park is artfully carved out of the densely forested hillside of Dorset Mountain.*

The first area you'll come to, Area A, has a pleasing mix of tent and lean-to sites, much like the rest of the campground. In the 1-through-12 section of the loop, most of the tent sites are set toward the center of the loop, with the lean-tos on the outside. For the most part, the lean-tos are secluded on the sides, with the open side of the lean-to facing out from the A-loop road.

The Willow lean-to and site 1 are small and adjacent to each other. Site 1 is secluded on the sides but open to the road. Willow is set a bit farther back, making it secluded. Cherry is fairly spacious and secluded, as it's set off the road in a dense grove of young maple and beech trees. Both the Pine and Hickory lean-tos are on smaller sites but feel moderately private.

Like the other tent sites in this part of the loop, site 5 is of moderate size but doesn't offer much privacy from the other sites. Site 6 is spacious and open to the road but is a bit more secluded than the other tent sites nearby. The Elm and Alder lean-tos are small and face the main campground road leading to the B and C areas, but they still feel secluded. Site 7 is open to the road but does have several large spruce trees growing up through it. Beech is a smaller site. It's close to the road but has a decent sense of seclusion, with beech trees (of course) peppering the site.

Poplar is on a good-sized site that is fairly private on the sides, but it's a bit open to the road. Site 8 is set up

RATINGS

Beauty: ☆☆☆☆☆
Privacy: ☆☆☆☆
Spaciousness: ☆☆☆☆
Quiet: ☆☆☆☆
Security: ☆☆☆☆
Cleanliness: ☆☆☆☆

ADDRESS:	65 Emerald Lake Lane East Dorset, VT 05253
OPERATED BY:	Vermont Agency of Natural Resources– Department of Forests, Parks, and Recreation
INFORMATION:	802-362-1655
OPEN:	Memorial Day– Columbus Day
SITES:	67 tent sites, 37 lean-to sites
EACH SITE:	Fire ring, picnic table
ASSIGNMENT:	First-come, first-served or by reservation: 888-409-7579, vtstateparks.com
REGISTRATION:	At ranger station at entrance to park
FACILITIES:	Day-use area, flush toilets, coin-operated showers, water spigots
PARKING:	At sites
FEE:	$16–$20 for tent sites, $23–$27 for lean-tos
RESTRICTIONS:	*Pets:* On leash only *Fires:* In fireplaces only *Alcohol:* At sites only *Vehicles:* Parking at sites only *Other:* Reservations require 2-night minimum stay; check in after 2 p.m., check out by 11 a.m.; quiet hours 10 p.m.– 7 a.m.; maximum 8 people per site

off the road but still has an open feel. It's encircled by slender beech trees and several large maples and spruce. The Spruce lean-to, as you may imagine, is set within a fairly dense spruce grove, although the lean-to itself is close to the road.

Locust is very spacious and offers an excellent sense of seclusion, set amid a loosely spaced grove of spruce. Larch is also spacious and secluded. It's way off the campground road within a shimmering, green grove of young beech trees. Birch is on a good-sized site and protected by a grove of spruce, although it's right on the corner of the campground road. It's also right next to the trail that leads to the lake.

The sites toward the end of Area A are more secluded and scenic. Site 15 is small but private and open to the sky. Site 16 is very sunny. It's a bit open and encircled by a loose forest of beech and spruce.

A line of spruce frames site 18, which is also spacious and has a canopy of beech overhead. A steep bank off to the right of the site leads down into a small ravine. Site 17 is moderate in size and secluded from the road by several large spruce trees. Site 19 is at the end of the loop. This site is fairly small, but it's nicely enshrouded by maples. It's just open enough to the sky so that plenty of sunlight filters down to the site.

Between the Area A loop and the B loop is a short strip containing sites 20 through 23. Even though they're far from the rest of the sites, they don't offer much seclusion from the road or from each other, but if you wanted some sites side-by-side, these would be just fine.

There's a campground host at site 27 (on the left as you enter Area B) and a small playground next to site 28. Nearby, site 29 and the Tamarack lean-to are both set up for wheelchair access. Both sites 32 and 34 abut the steep hillside behind them, which adds to the sense of seclusion. Site 36 is also isolated and set up against the hillside.

Sites 35, 37, 38, and 39 are in their own little neighborhood. These are spacious sites with a dark canopy of conifers. They're open to each other, but they make for a fantastic quartet of sites. A stone wall runs behind sites 38 and 39, which adds to their privacy. Of this group of sites, site 39 is probably the most secluded.

MAP

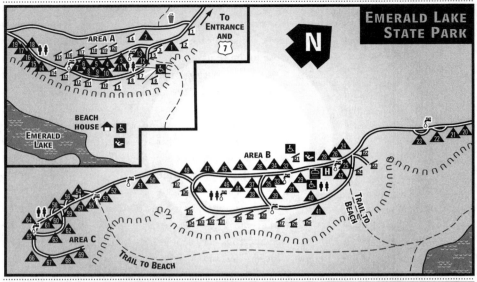

Sites 43 and 44 are across the road from each other but very well hidden on the sides from neighboring sites. Site 43 is also up against the hillside. Site 49 is spacious, fairly secluded, and set within a grove of young, slender maples. It also has the steep hill against its back, and a trail leading up Dorset Mountain is beside it.

Moving through the lower end of the B loop brings you to the lean-to sites. The Plum, Ginkgo, and Apple lean-tos are set in a trio. They're nicely secluded on the sides but set close to each other. A bit more road noise from US 7 is noticeable here, but only during the day. Dogwood is quite private, as it's set down off the road at the end of a longer driveway. Sumac is as well, although it's not quite as far off the road. Hazelnut, set off the road on a small rise, is enshrouded in a dark spruce grove.

GETTING THERE

From Interstate 91 north, take Exit 2 and follow VT 30 toward Manchester. Take US 7 north and follow this to the park.

GPS COORDINATES

N43° 17.047641'
W73° 0.181096'

There are two tent sites in here as well. Site 40 is huge. The bathroom building is behind it, but a small hill creates a sense of seclusion. It's also across from site 41, which is small but private. This site, too, is surrounded by small hills, almost as if it were landscaped, and nestled within a mixed forest of spruce and maples.

Farther up on this part of the loop, a trail leads down to the lake across from site 42 and the Sycamore lean-to. The sites and lean-tos here share the ambience of a waterfall in the background.

Moving into Area C, the Yew lean-to is on a small but private site. Sites 50 and 51 are close to each other but beautifully separated from the other sites in this part of the campground. They're both open to the sky and surrounded by young maple and beech trees. Sites 52 and 53 face the steep hill that runs along most of the northern side of the campground. They're open to the road but secluded on the sides. The trail leading down to Emerald Lake is right next to site 53.

As you head deeper into the Area C campsites, you'll find many that are rather small, not too private, and close to the restroom. But you'll also find some spacious and spectacularly secluded spots. Set up on a short loop of this part of the campground road and encircled by slender beech, maple, and birch, site 63 enjoys a shimmering green effect when the sun shines through the trees. It's open to this short loop but well secluded on the sides. Site 62 is a bit smaller and more hidden, surrounded by a picturesque mix of spruce and birch. Both of these sites are fairly close to the restroom but are set off by the stand of trees in the center of the loop.

As you near the far end of the campground road, you'll find site 66, which is an absolutely beautiful site surrounded by a grand mixed grove of mature beech, spruce, birch, and maple trees. It's open to the sky just enough for a glimpse of the sun and stars. Site 67 is also a large site surrounded by spruce for a cooler, shaded feel and a sense of seclusion. Sites 68 and 69 are at the absolute end of the campground road. They're fairly close to each other but marvelously private, carved out of dense spruce forest. These last few sites share that cool, dark, sylvan feeling. Emerald Lake State Park has many exquisite sites, but these more remote ones are among the best.

GIFFORD WOODS STATE PARK

GIFFORD WOODS IS A PERFECTLY SITUATED spot from which to launch your adventures into the Green Mountains and the Killington area. Whether you're here for late-season skiing or mountain biking at Killington or hiking in the Green Mountains (especially portions of the Appalachian Trail or Vermont's Long Trail), this is a great, centrally located base camp.

The Appalachian Trail passes right through the park, and it forms the right-hand border for site 12 within the campground. I happened to stay there one night and found it fascinating to be perched right on that fabled footpath. Turn left from this site and head for the summit of Katahdin; turn right for Amicalola Falls, Georgia.

As at other state-park campgrounds in Vermont, the site arrangement at Gifford Woods State Park is a loosely spaced combination of tent sites and lean-tos named for tree varieties. Two distinct areas exist within the campground: the Upper Loop and the Lower Loop. The whole upper area of the campground is set beneath a truly mixed woodland with deciduous and coniferous trees and old and new forest. Sites 1 and 2 are tucked in together right across from the playground, which is also off the Upper Loop's campground road. These are great if you need a pair of contiguous sites for a larger group. Conversely, you'll definitely meet your neighbors if you arrive previously unacquainted.

Site 3 is spacious, but it's right next to the playground, so it's not quite as private and could be noisy if there are a lot of kids on the swings and slide. This would be a great site to secure if you're camping with small kids and plan on spending time at the playground. Besides the playground, kids will like the footpath and self-guided nature tour that winds through the woods behind the playground and picnic area.

Sites 4 and 5 are well isolated, with a solid sense of privacy. Site 4 is pretty and private, even though it's set

> *Gifford Woods State Park is exceptional both as a relaxing destination and as a base camp for Green Mountain hiking adventures.*

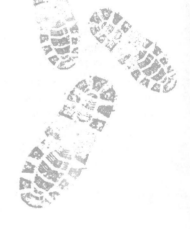

RATINGS

Beauty: ☆ ☆ ☆ ☆ ☆
Privacy: ☆ ☆ ☆ ☆
Spaciousness: ☆ ☆ ☆ ☆
Quiet: ☆ ☆ ☆ ☆
Security: ☆ ☆ ☆ ☆
Cleanliness: ☆ ☆ ☆ ☆

KEY INFORMATION

ADDRESS:	34 Gifford Woods Killington, VT 05761
OPERATED BY:	Vermont Agency of Natural Resources– Department of Forests, Parks, and Recreation
INFORMATION:	802-775-5354 (in season), 888-409-7579 (Oct.–May)
OPEN:	Mid-May–mid-Oct.
SITES:	22 tent sites, 20 lean-to sites, 4 cabins
EACH SITE:	Fire ring or brick hearth, picnic table
ASSIGNMENT:	First-come, first-served or by reservation: 888-409-7579, vtstate parks.com
REGISTRATION:	At ranger station
FACILITIES:	Coin-operated hot showers, flush toilets, playground, picnic area
PARKING:	At sites
FEE:	$16–$20 for tent sites, $23–$27 for lean-tos
RESTRICTIONS:	*Pets:* Dogs on leash only *Fires:* In fire rings only *Alcohol:* At sites only *Vehicles:* Parking at sites only *Other:* Reservations require 2-night minimum stay; check in after 2 p.m., check out by 11 a.m.; quiet hours 10 p.m.– 7 a.m.; maximum 8 people per site

right at the intersection where the one-way upper campground loop road rejoins itself. Site 5 is tucked off on its own in the woods, set back from the road.

Sites 6 and 7 are set a good distance off the road, but they're quite close to each other. Sites 9 and 10 are right across the campground road from each other. They're more open, so they aren't quite as private. Like sites 1 and 2, this pair would be fine for a group needing two sites.

Site 8 is fairly isolated, near the Ash lean-to. Site 11 isn't bad, but it's also a bit more open than some of the other sites in the Upper Loop. Site 11 is right across from the Appalachian Trail.

Aside from also being right on the Appalachian Trail, site 12 is otherwise another of Gifford Woods's top-notch tent spots. It has plenty of space and is fairly isolated. Site 13 is spacious and set back a bit from the road, but it has a water spigot nearby, so you'll get lots of visitors. If you want to meet a bunch of your campground neighbors, this is the site for you.

The lean-tos are interspersed among the tent sites. The Birch lean-to is in a pleasant, isolated spot. This one would be worth getting just for the privacy of the site. Apple and Maple are similarly off on their own.

Spruce is fairly isolated and on the inside of the loop. Hemlock is next to the frequently visited water spigot near site 13, but it's in the woods a ways, so it's more private. The Elm lean-to also has a decent distance between the site and the road.

Overall, the upper campground sites are quieter than the lower sites. The surrounding forest is thicker, and you're that much farther from VT 100. Still, there are some attractive spots on the lower loop as well. The lower loop includes sites 14 through 27.

Site 27, the first site you come to, is open and quite spacious, but consequently not very private. The same could be said about the first three lean-to sites within this loop: Oak, Walnut, and Poplar. The Willow, Aspen, and Cherry lean-tos are grouped close together as well. There aren't many trees between these sites. If you're having a camping family reunion or some other confluence of friends and family, securing either troika of lean-tos would give you the perfect venue.

MAP

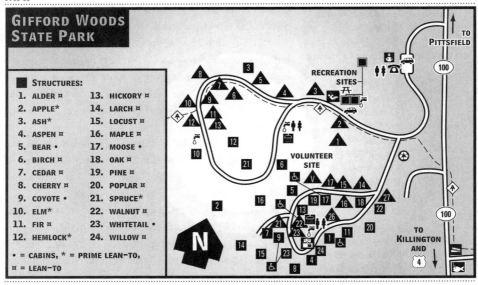

GIFFORD WOODS STATE PARK

STRUCTURES:

1. ALDER ¤	13. HICKORY ¤
2. APPLE*	14. LARCH ¤
3. ASH*	15. LOCUST ¤
4. ASPEN ¤	16. MAPLE ¤
5. BEAR •	17. MOOSE •
6. BIRCH ¤	18. OAK ¤
7. CEDAR ¤	19. PINE ¤
8. CHERRY ¤	20. POPLAR ¤
9. COYOTE •	21. SPRUCE*
10. ELM*	22. WALNUT ¤
11. FIR ¤	23. WHITETAIL •
12. HEMLOCK*	24. WILLOW ¤

• = CABINS, * = PRIME LEAN-TO,
¤ = LEAN-TO

The Fir lean-to is off on its own, right across from the restrooms. Site 26 is also conveniently located near the facilities, but it isn't very private. The Alder lean-to is set up for wheelchair access.

As you move farther along the loop and back into the tent sites, sites 21 through 23 are all moderately spaced and well isolated. Next to site 21, a short road leads up to another trio of lean-tos—Cedar, Locust, and Larch. If you have a very large group that wants to bunk out in a trio of lean-tos, Gifford Woods State Park is clearly where you want to be, specifically the Lower Loop, where most of the lean-tos are situated.

The woods around sites 15 through 17 are moderately dense. The sites also larger, so you'll run the risk of an RV dropping anchor next door. Similarly, site 14 is very open and has plenty of room to spread your wings (or your tarp and your tent's rainfly), but you'll give up a little privacy.

GETTING THERE

Gifford Woods State Park is right off VT 100, just north of the access road for Killington Resort.

GPS COORDINATES

N43° 40.597029'
W72° 48.629158'

Perhaps the nicest aspect of Gifford Woods State Park is that you don't have to travel far outside the park, or even inside the park, before you run across some hiking trails. As mentioned previously, the Appalachian Trail runs right through the park and reconnects with the Long Trail approximately 1.5 miles north of the park. Another spectacular sight to see is the 7-acre stand of old-growth hardwoods right across VT 100 from the campground. This pristine wilderness has some massive sugar maple, beech, birch, and ash trees. Tread lightly and enjoy this grand old forest.

THIS IS NO SANITIZED, DRIVE-IN, drive-out campground. The campsites at Grout Pond are spread out along a hiking trail that winds around the western shore of the pond. You have to hike your gear in to your tent site. This extra effort will give you a huge payoff, though.

You hike in to any of the 11 tent and lean-to sites via the Pond Loop Trail. This trail cuts through a dense forest, through which you can catch tantalizing glimpses of the pond as you start out. As its name implies, the Pond Loop Trail brings you all the way around Grout Pond. The campsites are spread liberally along the first mile of the trail. No camping is permitted beyond site 11, the last developed tent site. Since you hike in to the sites, parking is in the small lot past the campground host cabin.

Don't expect to happen upon the campsites as soon as you set out from the parking area. The first site is just under a 0.5-mile hike in. Carry a manageable amount of gear or, better yet, bring a wagon or some sort of wheeled cart to transport your stuff. If you're hauling gear without wheeled assistance, start out by bringing your tent to stake your claim on your site. These sites are first-come, first-served. Because you can't reserve them, it's a good idea to have a backup plan if they're full.

This is very rustic, primitive camping. These sites have a true wilderness feel that you'll usually experience only on backcountry backpacking trips.

At 0.1 mile down the Pond Loop, you'll come to a trailhead for the 3.2-mile East Loop, the 1-mile hike to the Kelley Stand parking area, and the 2-mile hike to the Somerset Reservoir. Shortly after passing this trailhead, you'll come to another trailhead for the Camp Loop, which follows a shorter loop out from the pond than the winding East Loop. Stay on the Pond Loop to get to the campsites.

> *These hike-in campsites give a sense of wilderness isolation you typically find only on extended backpacking trips—they are as remote as it gets.*

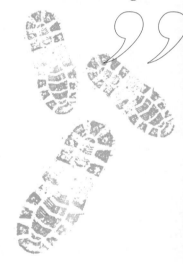

RATINGS

Beauty: ✩ ✩ ✩ ✩ ✩
Privacy: ✩ ✩ ✩ ✩ ✩
Spaciousness: ✩ ✩ ✩ ✩
Quiet: ✩ ✩ ✩ ✩ ✩
Security: ✩ ✩ ✩ ✩
Cleanliness: ✩ ✩ ✩ ✩ ✩

KEY INFORMATION

Site 1 is down off the trail, on the shore of Grout Pond. It's an incredibly spacious site where you'll get breezes blowing in off the pond and a decent amount of sunlight filtering through the moderately dense forest. The site is hidden in a very subtle way from the Pond Loop Trail by a stand of trees and a short stone wall. Down in the site, you'll have a clear view of the pond, and access to it for your canoe or kayak.

That brings up another point about getting to your site. Once you've marked your site with your tent, you could go back to your car and haul your gear in, taking four or five (or however many) trips. Or you could load up your canoe or kayak and paddle to the site. Then you've got your vessel right there at your campsite and you can explore the crystalline waters of Grout Pond after you've set up camp. You could also haul your gear inside your canoe or kayak atop a wheeled cart.

The next site on the Pond Loop Trail, site 2, is very isolated from the trail. Standing on the Pond Loop, you can barely see site 2. A twisting path leads down to the site, which is a bit smaller than site 1 but just as open to the pond, and extremely secluded.

If privacy is more important to you than being right on the pond, site 3 is a perfect choice. This site is set up in the woods away from the pond. You'll cross a series of short footbridges put there to minimize trail erosion. Please use the bridges—don't step off or around them. The site is set within a very dense forest of deciduous trees, with a lot of maple and beech. It's moderately spacious, but site 1 is clearly the largest at Grout Pond if that's an important factor.

Across the trail from the pond is site 4. Follow a 50-foot path up toward the site. It's a bit smaller than site 1 or 2 but is very nicely secluded.

Just past site 4 is a picnic area next to the pond. If you're waiting for someone to finish packing before you occupy a site, this is a great spot to rest and have a bite. When I first walked the Pond Loop, I mistook this for a campsite, but it's clearly marked as a no-camping and no-fires area.

Another superbly secluded site is 5, which is up in the woods on the opposite side of the trail from the pond. It gets dark early here, as very little evening sunlight

MAP

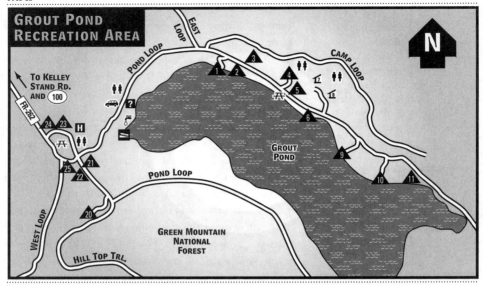

GROUT POND RECREATION AREA

EAST LOOP

POND LOOP

To KELLEY STAND RD. AND (100)

FR-262

CAMP LOOP

N

GROUT POND

POND LOOP

WEST LOOP

GREEN MOUNTAIN NATIONAL FOREST

HILL TOP TRL.

penetrates the extremely dense, mostly deciduous forest. The woods encircling site 5 afford campers a complete sense of solitude.

It may be fairly small, but site 6 is well isolated from the neighboring campsites. It's fairly small but has a tent platform, is very open to the sun, and is surrounded by a dense grove of young maple trees.

If you'd rather be way off in the woods, check out site 7. This lean-to site, accessed via a short hike off the main trail, is set within a grove of moderately spaced beech and ash trees and dense undergrowth. Site 8 is the other lean-to site, which is also set in the woods away from the pond. This one is in a fairly open part of the forest.

Sites 9, 10, and 11 are the farthest down the trail and the most-isolated sites. Site 9 is the first of these three gems and is set up so it faces Grout Pond. This is a perfect site for fishing or launching a canoe or kayak.

If ever there was a near-perfect site, it would have to be site 10, which is very isolated by virtue of its remote location on the Pond Loop and its distance from its nearest neighbors. A medium-sized site set beneath a loose stand of maples and spruce, it offers a nice, flat, grass-and-

GETTING THERE

From VT 100 in West Wardsboro, travel west on the Stratton–Arlington Road (a.k.a. Kelley Stand Road) for about 6 miles and turn left onto Forest Road 262 (look for the brown U.S. Forest Service sign). Follow FR 262 to the end.

GPS COORDINATES

N43° 2.825897'
W72° 57.092078'

moss-covered area for your tent carved out of the dense undergrowth. A tree hanging over the pond adds some character.

Site 11 affords a complete sense of isolation. It's on the pond side, about 70 feet from the Pond Loop Trail and distant from any neighbor. This is a moderately spacious site, set within a relatively dense forest of mostly deciduous trees and encircled by dense undergrowth to complete your wilderness camping experience.

These last couple of sites along the Pond Loop—sites 10 and 11—are as secluded and wild as just about any you will find in New England. The layout and character of site 10 make it my favorite. It has a Japanese-garden feel to it, with moss cover, artful spacing of the trees, one tree growing out over the pond, and an open flow. From site 10 you have a full view of the pond, and the openness allows you to enjoy the breezes and the sunlight, or the moonlight once dusk has fallen.

When you arrive at Grout Pond, you'll see some sites up near the campground host cabin, near the day-use area. These are likely spots for RVs. Pitch your tent here only as long as you have to wait for one of the pondside sites to open up.

THE CONTIGUOUS **B**OMOSEEN and Half Moon Pond state parks are essentially a string of ponds, marshlands, and abandoned quarry sites, all interconnected by several hiking trails ranging in length from 0.3 mile to 4.5 miles. From the sheltered enclave of Half Moon Pond, you could hike the Half Moon Pond Trail to the Glen Lake Trail, follow this through Beaver Meadow, and pass Moscow Pond to Glen Lake. From Glen Lake, the Slate History Trail will bring you to Lake Bomoseen.

The campground at Half Moon Pond State Park is divided into two areas along either side of the pond. The loop with sites 1 through 35 is off to the left as you enter the camping area, and the rest of the sites, 36 through 60, are off to the right. Both sides of the campground have sites perched right on the shore of Half Moon Pond. These are the best sites.

As you enter the 1-through-35 loop, sites 1 and 2 sit immediately on your left. They are spacious and set within a loose grove of maples and other deciduous trees. Situated right where the campground road splits, site 2 is very open.

Sites 4 and 6 both sit on the shore of Half Moon Pond. Site 4 is spacious and has a partially grass-covered surface upon which to pitch your tent. It's a bit close to site 6, which is on the left as you look at the pond. Still, this is a key spot if you've brought along a canoe or kayak. You could launch your boat right from your campsite. Site 6 is smaller than site 4, but it's also shadier. Paddlers and anglers should reserve sites 4 and 6, as they're perfectly suited for either activity.

Site 3 has a deeper sense of seclusion. It's up in the woods off the campground road, opposite but overlooking the pond. Site 5 is too open. The back side faces the restrooms, and the front opens to site 6.

The sites on the forest side of the campground loop road—sites 7, 10, and 11—are very spacious and open,

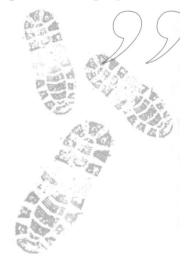

Half Moon Pond is pristine, and the campground that wraps around either side of it provides some spectacular pondside camping.

RATINGS

Beauty: ☆ ☆ ☆ ☆ ☆
Privacy: ☆ ☆ ☆ ☆
Spaciousness: ☆ ☆ ☆ ☆
Quiet: ☆ ☆ ☆ ☆ ☆
Security: ☆ ☆ ☆ ☆
Cleanliness: ☆ ☆ ☆ ☆

KEY INFORMATION

ADDRESS: 1621 Black Pond Rd. Fair Haven, VT 05743

OPERATED BY: Vermont Agency of Natural Resources– Department of Forests, Parks, and Recreation

INFORMATION: 802-273-2848 (summer), 888-409-7579 (Oct.–May)

OPEN: Memorial Day– Columbus Day

SITES: 53 tent sites, 11 lean-to sites, 5 cabins, 1 cottage

EACH SITE: Stone hearth, picnic table

ASSIGNMENT: First-come, first-served or by reservation: 888-409-7579, vtstate parks.com

REGISTRATION: At ranger station

FACILITIES: Coin-operated hot showers, flush toilets, water spigots, dump station

PARKING: At sites

FEE: $16–$20 for tent sites, $23–$27 for lean-tos

RESTRICTIONS: *Pets:* On leash only
Fires: In fire rings only
Alcohol: At sites only
Vehicles: Parking at sites only
Other: Reservations require 4-night minimum stay; check in after 2 p.m., check out by 11 a.m.; quiet hours 10 p.m.– 7 a.m.; maximum 8 people per site

but they still offer a bit of seclusion because they are surrounded by moderately dense deciduous forest. Sites 8, 9, 12, 13, and 14 are right on the pond but are bunched in close together. They are all super sites, separated by small stands of deciduous trees; however, they're smaller, more closely packed, and less private.

Site 15 is large and well isolated on the sides and back of the site, but it's open to the road. Sites 14 and 16 are right on the pond. Site 16, however, feels jammed in between the other sites. These open sites may not provide as much privacy, but then again, they're on the water. Site 17 is also right on the pond, but it's slightly larger, more private, and right next to the small beach area.

Sites 20 and 21 are well secluded on the sides, if not from the front. The Beaver lean-to is next to site 20. Site 19 is very open. It's also right next to the restrooms. Sites 23 and 24 have a similarly exposed character. These spacious sites are nestled within a grove of mixed hardwoods.

The 25-through-35 section of the loop generally gives you a choice between smaller pond side sites or larger, open, wooded sites. There's a cool, dark feel to the forest here, as the canopy is high and dense, but at the ground level, the campsites in the low 30s are very open. One plus in this section is a trailhead for the Nature Trail between sites 30 and 31.

Heading off to the right as you enter the campground brings you to its more secluded section, with sites 36 through 60. The boat-rental facility is also on this side of the pond. You'll find several fabulous pondside sites in this area. If you can, try to land in sites 48, 50, or 60—more on them in a moment.

The location of site 36 provides isolation on all sides. It's tucked into the contours of a small hill to the left of the campground road as you head in. There's no pond view, but it's spacious, scenic, and private. The hill on which site 36 is perched is in the center of a small loop where most of the lean-to sites are located, but you can't see them from the site. The seclusion of this site is marvelous.

There's a beautiful, open grove of pine trees across from site 38. The dark, slender pines poke up through the rich, brown carpet of pine needles, giving a silent, sylvan

MAP

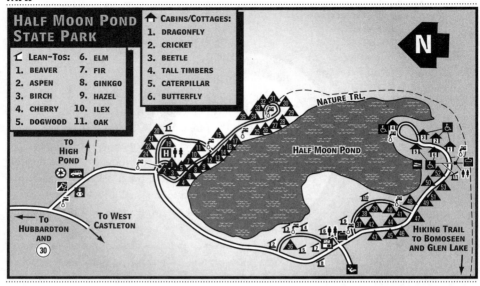

feel to this site. It's small but very well isolated. Site 37 shares a similar character, although it's a bit larger. It's also right across from the Hazel lean-to. Site 39 is small but secluded and right across from the Ilex lean-to.

Just outside site 40, across the road, a short footpath leads to the pond, so it's the next best thing to being on the water. Site 40 is also isolated and shady, set within a grove of young, mixed deciduous trees. Site 41 is narrow and on the small side, but it's carved out of a grove of young deciduous trees whose brilliant green leaves brighten the whole site.

Sites 42 and 43 sit opposite each other across the campground road. Site 42 is smaller and set in young mixed forest. Site 43 is very spacious and secluded on all sides, but it's open to the road and site 42. Sites 44 and 45 have a similar layout and arrangement. Site 44 is smaller than 45 and set within a grove of conifers and hardwoods. Site 45 is a little bigger and more secluded in a dense coniferous grove.

Site 46 is very spacious and secluded, set off the road in a dense, mixed forest. Sites 47 and 49 are moderately spacious but very open.

GETTING THERE

From VT 4 in Castleton Corners, take Exit 4 for VT 30 north. Follow this to Hubbardton. Turn left on Hortonville Road. Follow this to Black Pond Road. Turn left and follow this to the park.

GPS COORDINATES

N43° 41.930845'
W73° 13.343046'

The tradeoff of spaciousness and seclusion for a waterside setting is one I am usually quite willing to make. Site 48, for example, is small but right on the pond. There aren't many trees filling in the forest canopy directly overhead, so it has an open view to the sky and easy access to the water.

Site 50 is very spacious and provides a nice sense of seclusion. It's set among towering spruce trees right on the pond. While it's not on the pond and doesn't offer a clear pond view, site 51 does offer excellent seclusion, with dense forest on all sides. It's also up off the campground road.

Just before the boat-launch area is site 52, which is set within a spruce grove and is relatively roomy and private. Site 53 is a bit smaller than 52 and very open to the road. These sites are also near the boat-rental facility. You can rent a canoe for $5 an hour, $15 for a half-day, or $30 for a full day.

Dense undergrowth and a stand of trees isolate the cabin sites wrapped around the end of a short loop on the campground road. The Butterfly, Caterpillar, Beetle, Cricket, and Dragon-fly cabins and the Tall Timbers cottage are grouped together out here, within a grove of mixed deciduous and coniferous trees. Their best aspect is their location right on the pond.

Site 60 is also on this short loop. This site is large and set in a loose grove of spruce overlooking the pond. It's between the Tall Timbers cottage and the Caterpillar cabin.

36
JAMAICA STATE PARK

DON'T EVEN THINK OF COMING HERE without a reservation on one of the river-release weekends. When the West River swells to its banks, the campground at Jamaica State Park swells with whitewater kayakers.

If you want to score a site for one of those biannual weekends (one in the spring and one in the fall), you'll have to plan way ahead. Even for the rest of the year, Jamaica State Park's campground is heavily reserved. They do take first-come, first-served campers, but open sites can be hard to come by. Do yourself a favor and plan ahead for this one.

There are 41 tent sites and 18 lean-tos. Several lean-tos are arranged in a small loop at one end of the campground, but most sit in a line facing the West River. I can only imagine the scene during river-release weekends: lean-tos packed with camping and paddling gear and the river surging along, dotted with brilliantly colored kayaks and thrilled paddlers.

Generally, the campground and the surrounding park are very quiet. There are no major highways nearby, so there isn't much in the way of road noise. The campsites are situated beneath a forest of moderately spaced towering spruce and shorter, younger hardwoods. The dense undergrowth provides a nice sense of seclusion between most of the individual sites. The sites themselves are spacious and have a hard, sandy surface that's perfect for holding tent stakes.

The loop heading off to the right as you enter the camping area brings you to sites 1 through 11. There's a cathedral-like feel to the forest on this side of the campground, with the towering spruce trees presiding over the woodland. Sunlight and breezes flow easily through the forest to the sites.

Sites 1 and 2 are set back in the woods among the loosely spaced forest. Site 1 is open and fairly spacious. Site 2 is larger and set up off the campground loop

> *The atmosphere at Jamaica State Park mirrors that of the river: calm and serene most of the time, but wild when the whitewater is up.*

RATINGS

Beauty: ☆☆☆☆☆
Privacy: ☆☆☆☆
Spaciousness: ☆☆☆☆
Quiet: ☆☆☆☆
Security: ☆☆☆☆
Cleanliness: ☆☆☆☆

KEY INFORMATION

ADDRESS:	285 Salmon Hole Lane Jamaica, VT 05343
OPERATED BY:	Vermont Agency of Natural Resources–Department of Forests, Parks, and Recreation
INFORMATION:	802-874-4600 (summer), 888-409-7579 (Oct.–May)
OPEN:	Late April–Columbus Day
SITES:	41 tent sites, 18 lean-to sites
EACH SITE:	Fire ring, picnic table
ASSIGNMENT:	First-come, first-served or by reservation (strongly recommended): 888-409-7579, vtstateparks.com
REGISTRATION:	At ranger station
FACILITIES:	Hot showers, flush toilets, water spigots, playground
PARKING:	At sites
FEE:	$16–$20 for tent sites, $23–$27 for lean-tos
RESTRICTIONS:	*Pets:* On leash only *Fires:* In fire rings only *Alcohol:* At sites only *Vehicles:* Parking at sites only *Other:* Reservations require 4-night minimum stay; check in after 2 p.m., check out by 11 a.m.; quiet hours 10 p.m.–7 a.m.; maximum 8 people per site

road. It has an open feel that doesn't sacrifice its sense of privacy.

The added elevation of sites 3 and 4 makes them more secluded. These sites, roomy and clean, sit on a small rise off the campground loop road. Site 3 is opposite the volleyball net in the day-use area, which you can see through the woods. It's cool to be close to the action, but things could get noisy during the day. Site 4 is next to the restrooms. Site 5 is a little smaller than most of the other sites in this loop, but it's off the campground loop road, which adds privacy.

Nearby, the Briar lean-to is set up for wheelchair access. The rest of the lean-tos within this part of the loop face out from or are perpendicular to the loop road, which increases their privacy.

The lean-tos are spread out beneath the loosely spaced forest and against a good-sized hill that is peppered liberally with loosely spaced pine and spruce and coated in a soft blanket of pine needles. The effect is captivating. The Hackberry and Ironwood lean-tos are at the base of the hill. The forest is open enough here so that there's plenty of room to pitch tents at the lean-to sites.

A spruce grove and a small embankment give site 6 a pleasant sense of privacy from the lean-tos behind the site. However, site 6 is open to the Ironwood and Hackberry sites facing the hill. Site 7 is very spacious and airy but also secluded by a deep spruce grove and young deciduous trees on one side. This is helpful because it's also right next to the restrooms.

The added elevation of site 8 enhances its privacy. This spacious site is up on a platform off the campground road and surrounded by loosely spaced spruce and dense, young deciduous trees and undergrowth. Site 9 lies at the base of the hill next to the Juniper lean-to. This site is very isolated on both sides but open to site 8 across the road. Site 9 is large, and there's a handsome, open character to the forest here. Site 11 is roomy yet very secluded on all sides, framed by towering spruce trees. Site 10 also is spacious and private.

The campground loop is split by a short road, on which sites 12 and 13 are located. These sites are roomy but very exposed and close to the road. Site 12 is open to the sky, so the site itself receives lots of sunlight filtered

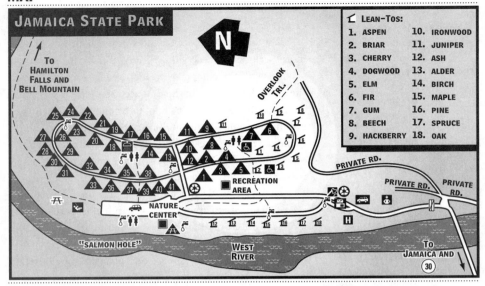

JAMAICA STATE PARK

N

To
HAMILTON
FALLS AND
BELL MOUNTAIN

OVERLOOK TRL.

PRIVATE RD.

PRIVATE RD.   PRIVATE RD.

RECREATION AREA

NATURE CENTER

"SALMON HOLE"

WEST RIVER

To
JAMAICA AND
30

Lean-Tos:

1.	ASPEN	10.	IRONWOOD
2.	BRIAR	11.	JUNIPER
3.	CHERRY	12.	ASH
4.	DOGWOOD	13.	ALDER
5.	ELM	14.	BIRCH
6.	FIR	15.	MAPLE
7.	GUM	16.	PINE
8.	BEECH	17.	SPRUCE
9.	HACKBERRY	18.	OAK

through the forest. The sites don't offer much in the way of privacy, though.

The forest is dense along the larger loop to the left as you enter the campground, which has sites 14 and up. The forest's character adds seclusion and privacy to these sites, most of which are moderately to very spacious. Site 14 is huge but doesn't provide much privacy, as it's very open on the sides. Sites 15 and 16 are both moderate in size and fairly well isolated.

Even though it's right across from the restrooms, site 17 has dense undergrowth on all sides. It's also set on a small rise, so it strikes a balance between moderate privacy and convenience to the facilities. Site 18 is spacious and open but not too private. Site 19 is a bit smaller and secluded on both sides, but it's open to the road.

Site 20 has a deep sense of privacy because it's down off the campground road. There's also a big rock in the center that you could use as a small table. This site is framed by spruce and dense undergrowth. Sites 21, 22, and 23 are all similar in size, shape, and spaciousness. Site 22 is off the campground road, and site 23 is down off the road. These are all fairly secluded and moderately spacious.

GETTING THERE

Follow VT 30 into Jamaica. Head east on Depot Street for 0.5 mile to the park.

GPS COORDINATES

N43° 6.286454'
W72° 46.366060'

Sites 24 and 25 are close together and a bit smaller than sites 21 through 23. Site 24 is set off the road a bit. Site 27 is huge but very open to the road. This site would be good for a larger group. Framed on the sides by dense undergrowth and spruce trees, it abuts the back of site 26. Site 29 is set down off the road and otherwise nicely secluded. It's very spacious and surrounded by dense, young undergrowth broken by towering spruce. Sites 28, 30, and 31 are similar in character in that they are moderately spacious and well isolated on the sides. Site 32 sits off the road in the dense undergrowth. It's smaller but nicely secluded.

If you're camping with kids, site 33 is a good choice, as it's right near the playground. It's also a great site if you plan to do a lot of hiking. A trailhead behind the playground leads you to the gentle, 2.5-mile Railroad Bed Trail, which follows the West River to the Ball Mountain Dam; the 2-mile Overlook Trail, which takes you up and over the summit of Little Ball Mountain; and the 3-mile Hamilton Falls Trail, which brings you to the dramatic 125-foot cascade of Hamilton Falls.

At sites 38 and above, the forest opens quite suddenly. These sites, separated by narrow stands of spruce and white pine, are roomy but open. It's up to you to decide how you feel about a site with this character, but I prefer sites that are more densely wooded.

There's a mixed sand-and-grass surface at site 39, which is framed by loose pines and spruce. This site is also right along the day-use parking area, separated by a relatively dense stand of trees.

Sites 39, 40, and 41 are all increasingly vast. These would work well for larger groups needing two or three contiguous sites. They're also great for stargazing or sunbathing, as they are wide open to the sky and they afford plenty of room to pile up paddling gear for those wild river-release weekends.

DIFFERENT PEOPLE ASSOCIATE Mount Ascutney with different things. For some, it may be the hiking. For a select group of people, hang gliding comes to mind. Mount Ascutney is one of the premier spots in New England from which to launch a hang glider. For those activities (well, at least the hiking and hang gliding), spending the night camped out in the state park at the base of Mount Ascutney is a great way to start.

There are two distinct camping areas within Mount Ascutney State Park. Sites 1 through 18 are off to the right as you enter the park. Sites 19 through 39 are in the loop off to the left. The auto road to the summit is directly ahead of you when you enter the park here.

I particularly like the sites in the 1-through-18 loop off to the right. They are spread out, so most provide solitude and seclusion. The forest here is a dense mix of primarily coniferous trees. The only caveat is that this side of the campground is fairly close to VT 44A, so you'll hear a bit of road noise during the day but not too much at night.

The first cluster of sites includes sites 1 through 5. The road on this side of the campground is a straight in-and-out, two-way road. The other side has a one-way loop. Site 1 is fairly small and right off the campground road. Site 2 is set off the road and more isolated. Sites 3, 4, and 5 are grouped together, but site 5 has a long driveway leading into it that adds to its privacy. Sites 3 and 4 would be good for a large group, as they are close together. The mixed forest gives the individual sites a shaded solitude.

Site 10 is spacious but open to the road and right across from the restrooms. Sites 9, 11, and 12 are set in a small group, much like sites 3, 4, and 5. Site 9 is too open and close to the road. Sites 11 and 12 are tucked around a corner off the campground road, so they offer a deeper sense of privacy. Again, all these sites are a stone's throw

> *Mount Ascutney has an elaborate network of hiking trails, easily accessible from the southern end of the campground.*

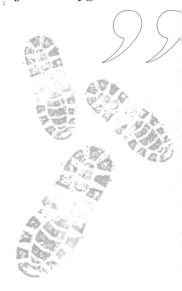

RATINGS

Beauty: ☆ ☆ ☆ ☆
Privacy: ☆ ☆ ☆ ☆
Spaciousness: ☆ ☆ ☆ ☆
Quiet: ☆ ☆ ☆
Security: ☆ ☆ ☆ ☆
Cleanliness: ☆ ☆ ☆ ☆

KEY INFORMATION

ADDRESS:	1826 Back Mountain Rd. Windsor, VT 05089
OPERATED BY:	Vermont Agency of Natural Resources–Department of Forests, Parks, and Recreation
INFORMATION:	802-674-2060 (summer), 888-409-7579 (Oct.–May)
OPEN:	Memorial Day–mid-Oct.
SITES:	39 tent sites, 10 lean-to sites
EACH SITE:	Stone hearth or fire ring, picnic table
ASSIGNMENT:	First-come, first-served or by reservation: 888-409-7579, vtstate parks.com
REGISTRATION:	At ranger station
FACILITIES:	Coin-operated hot showers, flush toilets, water spigots
PARKING:	At sites
FEE:	$16–$18 for tent sites, $23–$25 for lean-tos
RESTRICTIONS:	*Pets:* On leash only *Fires:* In fire rings only *Alcohol:* At sites only *Vehicles:* Parking at sites only *Other:* Reservations require 2-night minimum stay; check in after 2 p.m., check out by 11 a.m.; quiet hours 10 p.m.–7 a.m.; maximum 8 people per site

from VT 44A through the woods, so at times you will hear some road noise.

The next group of sites you'll encounter as you move down the campground road are sites 6 through 8. These three sites are also set in a cluster. Site 8 is near the restroom, which is a good thing for some people and not so good for others. Site 7 sits on a short spur off the campground road. Its added elevation gives it a little more privacy. These sites are all moderately spacious.

As you walk up to site 7, on your right you'll see the short footpath leading to site 6, which is very isolated, with about a 50-foot hike in to it. Site 6 has a fire ring instead of a hearth, which I generally prefer. Although the stone hearths are aesthetically pleasing, the iron fire rings seem to be safer, containing the fire, ashes, and coals on all sides.

The forest surrounding site 6 is relatively dense, but it thins directly above the site to let in lots of sunlight during the day and give you a clear view of the sky at night. Shadowy spruce trees spread out on all sides of the site, giving it a pleasant, dark, cool feel even on the warmest of summer days. There's still a bit of road noise from time to time, which is my only complaint about this otherwise excellent campsite.

A dense spruce grove with lots of fern ground cover surrounds site 13, so it offers a considerable sense of isolation while still being open to the road. Site 14 is small but down off the road, which makes it fairly secluded.

There's a small loop at the end of the campground road where sites 15 through 18 are located. A stand of towering spruce trees grows out of the center of the circle. Sites 15 and 16 are large but open to the road. Site 17, on a small rise above the campground road, is good-sized and fairly secluded. The best site within this loop is site 18. A path of about 25 feet leads up to it from its parking space. The site is set within a relatively dense grove of mixed deciduous and coniferous trees, but its distance from the road gives it an exquisite air of seclusion.

On to the other side of the campground: the second loop contains sites 19 through 39 and the lean-tos. Site 22 sits near the trailhead for the Futures Trail. From here you'll have access to a 1-mile hike to Bare Rock Vista, a

MAP

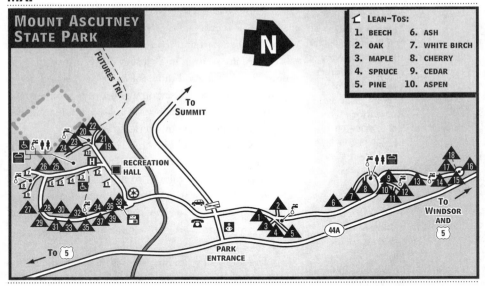

MOUNT ASCUTNEY STATE PARK

LEAN-TOS:

1. BEECH
2. OAK
3. MAPLE
4. SPRUCE
5. PINE

6. ASH
7. WHITE BIRCH
8. CHERRY
9. CEDAR
10. ASPEN

FUTURES TRL.

TO SUMMIT

RECREATION HALL

TO WINDSOR AND 5

44A

PARK ENTRANCE

TO 5

3.4-mile hike to the Steam Donkey overlook, a 4.1-mile hike to the junction with the Windsor Trail, and a 4.5-mile hike to the summit of Mount Ascutney.

Site 22 has a solitary quality, roomy and buffered on all sides by woods. I like this site the best on this side of the campground. Site 21 is also very spacious, but the side of site 21 is the back of site 19. You can see right through one site to the other. Site 20 is spacious and more open than these two, and it's set within fairly dense forest. The arrangement of sites 19 and 21 makes them a good pair for a group.

A low canopy of spruce trees adds to the solitude at site 23. It's a bit small, though. Site 24 is tucked off to the left, and it's also isolated on the sides, but it opens in the back to the sites behind it and to the lean-tos set around an open area. Most of the lean-tos at Mount Ascutney State Park sit in an open field and a loose grove of spruce and maple. The Oak and Beech lean-tos are the most exposed and the least private. The Maple lean-to is set up for wheelchair access and is right across from the

GETTING THERE

Take I-91 to Exit 8. From there, follow US 5 almost 2 miles to VT 44A. Follow VT 44A about 1 mile until you see signs for the park.

GPS COORDINATES

N43° 26.263883'
W72° 24.345374'

restroom and the campground host site. The Pine lean-to is nicely isolated and set within a tall grove of spruce.

Sites 25 and 26 are both moderately spacious and set within a loosely spaced grove of spruce with dense undergrowth. These two sites are secluded on the sides but somewhat open to each other. The White Birch and Cherry lean-tos lie at the end of a short spur off the campground road. They are close to each other but great for a larger group.

A grove of maples and other mixed deciduous varieties surrounds the spacious site 27, which is open to the sky and set off the campground road. Sites 29 and 31 are spacious but open to the road. You'll still hear occasional road noise from VT 44A on this side of the campground, especially in this part of the loop.

Set back from the campground road, sites 28 and 30 feel isolated, and site 30 is exceptionally spacious. Site 33 is open to the road but separated from neighboring sites. A loose grove of spruce borders the back of the site, and a wall of deciduous trees and dense undergrowth defines the sides. A short footpath right next to this site takes you to the playground area and the restroom.

A slightly longer entryway leads to site 35, buffering it from the campground road. Sites 34 and 37 are across the road from each other but buffered on either side. Site 34 is moderately spacious, while site 37 is huge and very open above.

Site 36 is just like site 34 in size and shape. Site 38 is also similar, but it's a bit larger and very open to the sky. Site 39 is set off the campground road, making it private. It's also set within a dense grove of mixed conifers and hardwoods with lots of underbrush.

Whether it's the hiking or the hang gliding that brings you to Mount Ascutney State Park, a night in one of the campground's secluded sites will be a night well spent.

WANT TO FEEL LIKE you're really getting away from it all? Moosalamoo Campground offers an incredibly remote wilderness atmosphere. To get to the campground, you turn off the paved road (actually US 7), and start heading down a long and winding dirt road. This is called the Goshen Road, as it will eventually lead you to the town of Goshen. Several miles down on the right, you'll come to the road leading into the campground. If our campground ratings judged seclusion, this would easily get six stars.

Moosalamoo is the Abenaki Indian word thought to mean "the moose departs" or "he trails the moose." The Abenakis frequently traveled through and stayed in this region, and their history and legacy linger.

The entire campground and all the campsites within are shaded by a mixed forest of hardwoods, with lots of maple and birch. The brilliant green leaves at the height of spring and summer cast a glow over the campground. The forest is young and spaced loosely enough to let generous amounts of light reach the campsites.

Moosalamoo has a total of 18 sites set on both sides of the short campground loop road. The sites are large and spaced well apart with plenty of room at each to accommodate the group limit of eight campers per site. Moosalamoo Campground would also score six stars for site spaciousness if the scale in this book went that high!

The campground host is in site 1, which is off to the left as you enter the campground loop. Behind site 1, you'll catch your first glimpse of the big, open field in the center of the campground. There's also a little arboretum out there with a variety of deciduous and coniferous trees. The sign in front of the arboretum calls it a Backyard Wildlife Habitat. The evergreens within were planted in memory of former campground hostess Sarah Foster.

> *When you're camping at Moosalamoo Campground, you are truly out in the wilderness.*

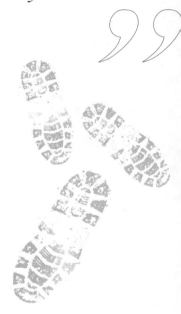

RATINGS

Beauty: ☆☆☆☆☆
Privacy: ☆☆☆☆☆
Spaciousness: ☆☆☆☆
Quiet: ☆☆☆☆☆
Security: ☆☆☆☆
Cleanliness: ☆☆☆☆

KEY INFORMATION

ADDRESS:	Forest Road 24 Ripton, VT 05766
OPERATED BY:	Green Mountain National Forest
INFORMATION:	Middlebury Ranger District, 1007 VT 7 South, Middlebury, VT 05753-8999; 802-388-4362
OPEN:	Memorial Day–Labor Day
SITES:	18
EACH SITE:	Fire ring, picnic table
ASSIGNMENT:	First-come, first-served
REGISTRATION:	Pay at self-serve fee station
FACILITIES:	Pit toilets, hand water pumps
PARKING:	At sites
FEE:	$10
RESTRICTIONS:	*Pets:* On leash only *Fires:* In fire rings only *Alcohol:* At sites only *Vehicles:* Maximum 2 per site *Other:* Check out by 2 p.m.; quiet hours 10 p.m.–6 a.m.; maximum 8 people per site; 14-day maximum stay; Green Mountain National Forest is closed to ATVs (woo-hoo!)

As you get deeper into the campground loop past site 4, the forest becomes denser and the sites feel even wilder and more isolated. Sites 7, 9, 11, and most of the other odd-numbered sites on the inner side of the campground loop are set against the central open field. If you camp on one of the inner loop sites, you'll be able to walk out the back of your site into this field, which is perfect for a game of Frisbee, lying in the sun, or stargazing.

Most of the sites are fairly uniform in size, but sites 10 and 14 are extra-large. They each have two picnic tables. Site 16 and 17 are pretty big as well but are equipped with only one table apiece. Any of these are worth investigating if you're camping with a larger group or family. Site 19 is right next to the arboretum, a pleasant aspect. It's also quite close to the recycling station.

Moosalamoo Campground is small and intimate, with a wonderful sense of remoteness. I can think of only one caveat, although it certainly isn't unique to this campground: bring whatever bug spray works best for you. You'll be deep in the woods here, and the insects can be ravenous.

Plenty of hiking trails lie within easy reach of the campground. You'll see trailheads for the Mount Moosalamoo and North Branch trails as you enter. The blue-blazed trails are the local hiking trails. The white-blazed trails are the Appalachian Trail and the Long Trail, which overlap through the Moosalamoo region.

There's also a trailhead right outside the campground for the Voter Brook Overlook.

All of these trails intersect other trail networks that wind throughout the forest in this part of Vermont. Try to get your hand on a trail map, because the trail network is extensive, and it wouldn't be too difficult to wander off a bit farther than you intended.

MAP

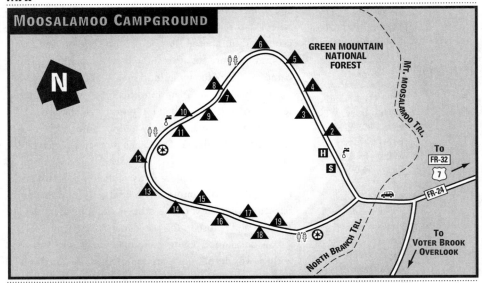

MOOSALAMOO CAMPGROUND

N

GREEN MOUNTAIN
NATIONAL
FOREST

6
5
8
7
4
10
9
3
11
2
12
H
S
13
15
14
16 17
18 19

Mt. MOOSALAMOO TRL.

To
FR-32
7

FR-24

NORTH BRANCH TRL.

To
VOTER BROOK
OVERLOOK

GETTING THERE

Follow US 7 west, past
Middlebury College's Snow
Bowl and its Bread Loaf
campus. Turn left on Forest
Road 32 (Goshen Road).
Follow this dirt road 3.3 miles
and turn right on FR 24.

GPS COORDINATES

N43° 55.113158'
W73° 1.531777'

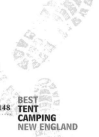

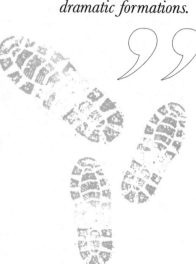

> *There are numerous short hikes in and around Quechee Gorge—you could spend countless hours gazing up into the dramatic formations.*

IN A STATE FULL OF incredible natural spectacles, Quechee Gorge has got to be one of Vermont's most amazing and unique sights. Plunging 165 feet down to the Ottauquechee River—whew, I'm glad they shortened that to name the gorge—Quechee Gorge reminds me of the scene in *Butch Cassidy and the Sundance Kid* where Robert Redford and Paul Newman, when cornered by the "good" guys, jump off their perch on a sheer cliff into a raging river.

Seen from the US 4 bridge that passes over it, the gorge's depth looks almost surreal. You'll be able to tell when you're there, even if you miss the signs for the gorge and the state park. There are always a bunch of people who have stopped to look over the bridge.

Just before you get to the gorge (if you're heading north on US 4), you'll come to the campground at Quechee State Park, tucked quietly off on the left opposite the tourist shops selling T-shirts and maple syrup on the other side of the road. For the most part, the campground is in a loosely spaced forest of conifers without much undergrowth. That factor, combined with the spacing and height of trees, gives the forest a statuesque presence. Visitors feel protected and secluded beneath the forest canopy. The spicy scent of coniferous trees, mixed in with the musty aroma of wood smoke, brings you instantly into the deep wilderness. Olfactory delights abound here.

Overall, the sites are large and somewhat open. You could land a space shuttle in site 2, yet it still feels fairly isolated from the neighboring sites by the forest and a bit of undergrowth. You'll hear some road noise from nearby US 4, but it's not too bad. At night, it's guaranteed to lessen. Also, the road noise is reduced the farther back you go in the campground, and it fades to nearly nothing at night.

Site 6 is right across from the restroom and shower building. A small playground sits behind the restroom

RATINGS

Beauty: ✩ ✩ ✩ ✩ ✩
Privacy: ✩ ✩ ✩ ✩
Spaciousness: ✩ ✩ ✩ ✩
Quiet: ✩ ✩ ✩
Security: ✩ ✩ ✩ ✩
Cleanliness: ✩ ✩ ✩ ✩

building. Whether or not you want to be close to these is your call.

A steep embankment falls away from the campground behind sites 7 through 14. This is not part of Quechee Gorge per se, but perhaps the river flowed this way many moons ago. This feature of the landscape makes for dramatic scenery, but you'll need to be extra-cautious if you have kids running around. A tumble down this embankment would be grim.

The Birch lean-to is also along the steep drop-off by sites 7 through 14.

Site 9 is huge and shielded overhead by the forest canopy, although it's very open at the ground level. You find these same characteristics at sites 12 and 10. These two sites are also close to each other, which is particularly appealing for a larger group that might want two adjoining sites.

The Walnut and Ash lean-tos are right next to each other, also a good pair for a group large enough to need two. The Hickory and Hackberry lean-tos are also adjacent. The lean-tos in the Vermont state-park campgrounds being named for tree varieties, a new species is just one more thing you might learn while camping here.

Another good pair of sites for a larger group would be 18 and 19. These two are very open and close together. What these sites lack in privacy they make up for in spaciousness. Quite close to a large, open field in the center of the campground, these are good sites for those camping with a tribe of kids who need a place for them to run around and burn off some of their seemingly boundless energy. The swing set and slides are in this field. There is also a trailhead for the Quechee Gorge Trail at the nearby intersection of the campground roads. This short trail is perfect for a quick walk after dinner.

Set against the woods bordering the central field, sites 20 and 21 are moderately spacious and allow easy access to the field. The Pine lean-to is also on the field. It's very open and not too private, but it is configured for disabled access. The campground also winds around a bit closer to US 4 here, so the proximity to the road and the field can make things a bit noisy.

There will be road noise at sites 23 through 28. Site 23 is huge but wide open. This site is also right next to

KEY INFORMATION

ADDRESS:	764 Dewey Mills Rd. White River Junction, VT 05001
OPERATED BY:	Vermont Agency of Natural Resources–Department of Forests, Parks, and Recreation
INFORMATION:	802-295-2990 (summer), 888-409-7579 (Oct.–May)
OPEN:	Memorial Day–mid-Oct.
SITES:	45 tent sites, 7 lean-to sites
EACH SITE:	Fire ring, picnic table
ASSIGNMENT:	First-come, first-served or by reservation: 888-409-7579, vtstate parks.com
REGISTRATION:	At ranger station
FACILITIES:	Coin-operated hot showers, flush toilets, playground
PARKING:	At sites
FEE:	$16–$20 for tent sites, $23–$27 for lean-tos
RESTRICTIONS:	*Pets:* On leash only *Fires:* In fire rings only *Alcohol:* At sites only *Vehicles:* Parking at sites only *Other:* Reservations require 2-night minimum stay; check in after 2 p.m., check out by 11 a.m.; quiet hours 10 p.m.–7 a.m.; maximum 8 people per site

MAP

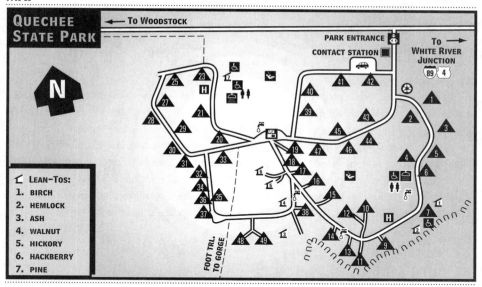

QUECHEE STATE PARK

← To Woodstock

PARK ENTRANCE
CONTACT STATION
To → WHITE RIVER JUNCTION
89 4

LEAN-TOS:
1. BIRCH
2. HEMLOCK
3. ASH
4. WALNUT
5. HICKORY
6. HACKBERRY
7. PINE

FOOT TRL. TO GORGE

GETTING THERE

From I-89 in Vermont, follow US 4 north toward the town of Quechee. The signs for the campground are right before Quechee Gorge itself.

GPS COORDINATES

N43° 38.226199'
W72° 24.036148'

part of the Quechee Gorge Trail, which is a mere 0.21 mile away. Site 27 is open, spacious, and set within a spruce grove. Site 29 is spacious and open, but the back of the site opens to the field. Site 30 is set within a grove of mixed deciduous and coniferous trees. This site faces the gorge, so through openings in the forest, there's a view as the gorge drops away below. Site 31 is spacious and set beneath a coniferous grove, so the floor is covered with a blanket of pine needles and leaves upon which you can pitch your tent.

A steep drop-off faces sites 31 through 37. The scenery is nothing short of dramatic, but you have numerous additional reasons to keep a close eye (or a short leash) on the kids. Sites 32 and 34 are quite open and spacious, but not as private as the rest. Site 35 is very open. The back of the site opens to the back of the lean-to sites.

At the end of this spur off the campground loop, site 37 is set in a quiet grove of conifers and offers a nice sense of isolation. It's an incredible campsite: spacious, framed by conifers, and open to the sky for lots of sunlight. Site 37 is also right next to the Quechee Gorge Trail, which is a short hike down to the gorge from the campground.

Site 38 sits between the Walnut and Ash lean-tos. It's framed by dense woods but is very open in front. Within the 42-through-47 loop, site 47 is huge and somewhat open in front and above, but it has dense forest on the sides.

Sites 48 and 49 are fairly close together and share an entry off the campground road. Site 48 is a bit farther off the road. Both sites are also right near the hiking trail leading to the gorge.

Site 45, set within a pine grove, is also huge and has an open feel. Sites 44 and 46 are a bit smaller but still have a nice isolated feel. Site 43 is huge and open. This site is also set within a grove of pines but is a bit closer to the road and the recycling station.

It's a bit smaller than some of its neighbors, but site 39 is quite spacious nonetheless. This site is carved out of a grove of loosely spaced white pines. Site 40 is open and spacious and set within loosely spaced pines. It's a beautiful site, but it's also on the US 4 side of the campground, so you'll hear some road noise. Sites 42 and 43 are a bit more open and also closer to the campground loop road, so they're not as quiet as Quechee's more secluded sites.

> *Settled high in the Green Mountains, Smugglers Notch Campground has a quiet, secluded feel and easy access to some of the best hiking in Vermont.*

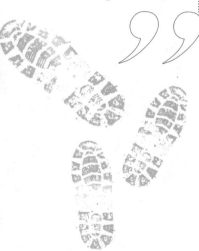

EVER WONDER WHERE THE "SMUGGLERS" in Smugglers Notch comes from? Me too. Apparently, when President Thomas Jefferson passed an embargo forbidding trade with Great Britain and Canada in 1807, it was especially hard on the folks living in northern Vermont. Most of those industrious, independent Vermonters kept right on trading with Montreal, moving cattle and other goods up through the narrow passage between the towering 1,000-foot cliffs. They established a grand tradition of smuggling that continued with abolitionists helping slaves head north to seek liberation in Canada and rumrunners bringing liquor south into the country from Canada during Prohibition.

These days, things are a bit quieter in the notch. The campground at Smugglers Notch State Park is across the road from part of Stowe Mountain Resort ski area, so you get glimpses of the towering mountain through the trees. You're also surrounded by Mount Mansfield State Forest, so the hiking opportunities are virtually limitless. The campground is in a mixed, mostly deciduous forest, with an open field in the center. It's very quiet, especially at night, and even during the warmest periods of summer, the air is crisp and cool this high up in the Green Mountains.

The sites at Smugglers Notch are clustered on the inside and outside of the campground loop road. There are also a handful of hike-in sites on the outside of the road. The rangers have labeled the tent sites and lean-to sites as Prime or Regular. When you're choosing your site, you can safely follow their assessments. Hermit Island in Maine does a similar thing, ranking sites by location and seclusion.

Most of the lean-to sites on the inside of the loop—Ash, Elm, Beech, and Maple—surround a small open area and loosely spaced trees. Except for Elm, these are labeled as Regular lean-to sites. Also in the lower half of

RATINGS

Beauty: ☆ ☆ ☆ ☆ ☆
Privacy: ☆ ☆ ☆ ☆
Spaciousness: ☆ ☆ ☆ ☆
Quiet: ☆ ☆ ☆ ☆ ☆
Security: ☆ ☆ ☆ ☆
Cleanliness: ☆ ☆ ☆ ☆

the loop are tent sites 3, 19, and 20. Site 20 is considered a Prime site, and it does offer privacy even though it's fairly close to the restrooms.

Tent sites 1 and 2 are nicely secluded from each other and from the road. They're down off the bottom of the campground loop a short hike from the road. You will hear some sporadic road noise from VT 108 on this end of the campground loop, but it fades to practically nothing at night.

Most of the rest of the lean-to sites are on the outside of the campground loop road. These include the Pine, Hemlock, Spruce, Balsam, and Oak sites. Balsam and Pine are considered Prime lean-to sites, and indeed they are set back a bit farther from the road to offer more privacy. Oak is a wheelchair-accessible lean-to site. Tent site 4, which is nearby, is also a wheelchair-accessible site.

The small "village" of hike-in tent sites, including sites 5, 6, 8, 9, 11, 12, and 13, are interspersed with the Larch, Cedar, and Aspen lean-to sites. Short hike-in trails lead into all of these sites, and a longer trail interconnecting the sites runs roughly parallel to the campground road. This is a nice collection of spots within a relatively loosely spaced forest of mixed deciduous and coniferous trees.

At the top of the campground loop road, farthest from the ranger station, are most of the Prime tent sites. Sites 7, 10, 14, and 15 are on the inside of the campground loop road and are all rightfully considered Prime sites. The Birch lean-to site is next to site 15. The forest here is a mixed, mostly deciduous forest with lots of beech, birch, and maple. On bright, sunny days, the forest seems to glow green, and at night it offers seclusion for the tent sites.

Sites 16, 17, and 18 are hike-in sites well off to the outside of the campground road. These are some of my preferred spots (and are indeed considered Prime sites), as they offer a delightful sense of seclusion. The Cherry lean-to is also off on its own just past site 16. Generally speaking, the Prime sites—whether you opt for a tent or a lean-to—are worth the extra couple of bucks. The sense of seclusion you'll gain from scoring one of these sites is well worth it.

KEY INFORMATION

ADDRESS: 7248 Smugglers Notch Rd. Stowe, VT 05672

OPERATED BY: Vermont Agency of Natural Resources– Department of Forests, Parks, and Recreation

INFORMATION: 802-253-4014 (summer), 800-658-6934 (January–May)

OPEN: Mid-May–mid-Oct.

SITES: 20 tent sites and 14 lean-to sites

EACH SITE: Stone hearth and picnic table

ASSIGNMENT: First-come, first-served or by reservation: 888-409-7579, vtstate parks.com

REGISTRATION: At ranger station

FACILITIES: Hot showers, flush toilets

PARKING: At sites

FEE: $16–$20 for tent sites, $23–$27 for lean-tos

RESTRICTIONS: *Pets:* On leash only
Fires: In established fireplaces only
Alcohol: At sites only
Vehicles: Parking at sites only
Other: Check in after 2 p.m., check out by 11 a.m., quiet hours 10 p.m.–7 a.m.; maximum 8 people per site; 2-day minimum stay for reservations

MAP

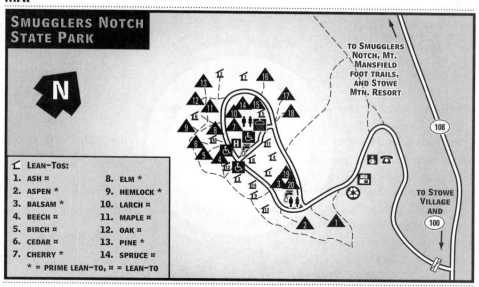

SMUGGLERS NOTCH STATE PARK

N

TO SMUGGLERS NOTCH, MT. MANSFIELD FOOT TRAILS, AND STOWE MTN. RESORT

108

TO STOWE VILLAGE AND 100

LEAN-TOS:

1. ASH ¤	8. ELM *
2. ASPEN *	9. HEMLOCK *
3. BALSAM *	10. LARCH ¤
4. BEECH ¤	11. MAPLE ¤
5. BIRCH ¤	12. OAK ¤
6. CEDAR ¤	13. PINE *
7. CHERRY *	14. SPRUCE ¤

* = PRIME LEAN-TO, ¤ = LEAN-TO

GETTING THERE

Follow VT 100 north to VT 108. Follow VT 108 past Stowe Mountain Resort to the state park, on the right and across the road from the northeastern part of the ski area.

GPS COORDINATES

N44° 31.211329'
W72° 46.278841'

Camping at Smugglers Notch puts you right across the road from Mount Mansfield. This is Vermont's highest peak and home to some of the world-class hiking for which Vermont is renowned. Thirty-five miles of hiking trails wind up and over Mount Mansfield, so plan your hike and pay attention. It wouldn't do to inadvertently come down on the other side of the mountain.

Test yourself on classics like the aptly named Profanity Trail and Subway, or you can opt for any of a variety of routes that connect to the Long Trail. Even below the summit, this ridgeline hike passes by overlooks with stunning views of the Green Mountains.

THE AIR IS CLEAR AND COOL as you approach Underhill State Park. Perched on the western flanks of Mount Mansfield, Vermont's highest peak, this is the best place from which to launch your hiking adventures on and around this renowned peak. You can literally begin a hike up Mount Mansfield from your campsite.

Underhill State Park itself feels remarkably isolated. At night, the silence and solitude are complete, the darkness absolute. Most of the sites are hike-ins, which adds to the sense of seclusion.

Sites 8 through 11 are farthest from the rest of the campground. These hike-in sites are up past the park shelter, an open log-cabin-type structure in the day-use and picnic area. The sites all require a hike of between 50 and 70 feet, so they are well secluded. The only other people you'll see from within one of these sites are your immediate neighbors, and at night all you'll see are glimmers of their campfire through the moderately dense forest of mostly young deciduous trees, with lots of beech and maples. Sites 8 through 11 aren't especially large, especially since much of the center is occupied by the large stone hearth. However, their sense of solitude more than makes up for their modest size.

There is a separate parking area for these hike-in sites, so you won't have to lug your gear quite as far as if you'd parked down by the park office. This parking area is also used by day-hikers going up Mount Mansfield, so if it's full when you first arrive, be patient and try again later.

Across the campground road from this small parking area is the Pine lean-to, which is also accessed via a short hike. It would be worth getting this site just for its sense of seclusion. You won't see anyone or anything but the surrounding deciduous forest.

You can also get to sites 8 through 11 by hiking up past the park shelter. On the way up to site 9, you'll pass

> *Underhill State Park's campsites are mostly hike-in sites. This design and its remote mountainside location add to the campground's wilderness feel.*

RATINGS

Beauty: ☆ ☆ ☆ ☆ ☆
Privacy: ☆ ☆ ☆ ☆
Spaciousness: ☆ ☆ ☆ ☆
Quiet: ☆ ☆ ☆ ☆ ☆
Security: ☆ ☆ ☆ ☆ ☆
Cleanliness: ☆ ☆ ☆ ☆ ☆

KEY INFORMATION

ADDRESS: P.O. Box 249
Underhill Center,
VT 05490

OPERATED BY: Vermont Agency of
Natural Resources–
Department of
Forests, Parks, and
Recreation

INFORMATION: 802-899-3022 (summer) or 800-252-2363 (Jan.–May)

OPEN: Memorial Day–mid-Oct.

SITES: 11 tent sites,
2 group sites,
13 lean-to sites

EACH SITE: Stone hearth,
picnic table

ASSIGNMENT: First-come, first-served or by
reservation: 888-409-7579, vtstate
parks.com

REGISTRATION: At ranger station

FACILITIES: Flush toilets, water

PARKING: At either of 2 central parking areas

FEE: $16–$18 for tent
sites, $23–$25 for
lean-tos

RESTRICTIONS: *Pets:* On leash only
Fires: In established
fire rings only
Alcohol: At sites only
Vehicles: Parking in
either of 2 small
lots near groups of
sites
Other: Check in
after 2 p.m., check
out by 11 a.m.;
quiet hours 10
p.m.–7 a.m.; maximum 8 people
per site; 2-day
minimum stay for
reservations

a water spigot. Fortunately, the site itself is farther up the trail, so you won't have people just walking by on the way to fill their canteens and hydration packs for the hike up Mansfield.

I love these kinds of hike-in sites because they really add to the wilderness feel. Wheeled carts are available by the ranger station to help you haul your gear into the sites. Sites 6 and 7 are also hike-in sites, spread out along a walking path that winds out from the ranger station in a short loop. These two sites are a bit larger than sites 8 through 11. Site 7 is moderately spacious but fabulously shrouded in dense forest.

Site 6 feels isolated. It has a short wooden retaining wall that keeps the tent platform intact and level. Set beneath a grove of tall spruce trees, it has a deep, woodsy, cool feel. The forest is loosely spaced enough that it lets lots of sunlight. This too adds to the unique character of this site. It's relatively close to the restrooms, but not too close.

The Cedar lean-to, on the other hand, is right behind the bathroom building—a bit too close for my taste. Site 5 and the Ash lean-to are also tucked in down behind the Cedar lean-to. Site 5 is set within a moderately dense forest at the edge of the woods and open area in which the Cedar lean-to is situated. Site 5 and the Ash lean-to are at the edge of a fairly steep bank as well, which adds to the character of the sites but requires you to be extra-cautious if you're camping here with kids.

An open, grassy area sits right across the parking lot from the ranger station. Sites 1 through 4 and the Maple, Birch, and Beech lean-tos surround this small field. These sites are a bit too exposed, but it's so quiet and dark here at night that it wouldn't matter much as evening fell. These sites also face a steep embankment.

Off to the left at the edge of the picnic area is tiny site 4. You'd have trouble pitching a tent designed for more than two people here. Sites 1 through 3 are moderately spacious and a bit more set off. Site 1 sits a bit higher up than the others. All three are carved out of fairly dense forest surrounding the open field and the picnic area. Since all of the other sites here are hike-in sites, these are the most easily accessible.

MAP

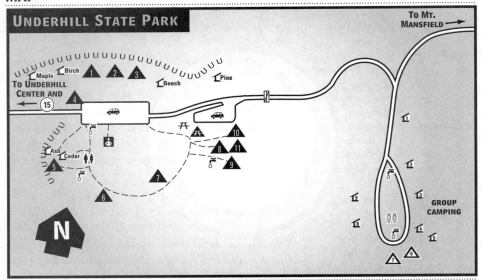

Wherever you land at Underhill State Park, you won't be far from the trails that follow the spine of the Green Mountains and bring you to the highest point in Vermont.

GETTING THERE

Follow VT 15 to Underhill Center. Turn onto Pleasant Valley Road. Follow this through the town of Underhill to Mountain Road. Turn onto Mountain Road and follow the signs to the park.

GPS COORDINATES

N44° 31.744924'
W72° 50.585890'

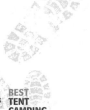

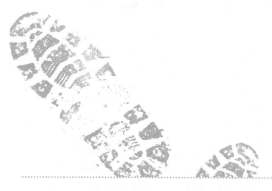

MASSACHUSETTS

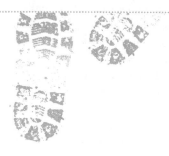

42
BEARTOWN
STATE FOREST

BEARTOWN STATE FOREST is home to a beautiful, intimate campground set along the shores of Benedict Pond, a good-sized body of water ready to accept anglers, swimmers, and paddlers. The campground has only 12 sites, but if there were a rating for perfect sites, Beartown would be way out in front.

Camping here is by reservation only (in season), so plan ahead, call ahead, and try to get yourself one of the spectacularly scenic pondside sites. The Appalachian Trail passes right through the forest and next to the campground. If I were hiking the Appalachian Trail, I would think it worth the effort to plan for a night at Beartown State Forest—especially if I could secure site 11.

Sites 1 and 2 are spacious. Site 1 is huge, in fact, with a large, grassy area where you could place your tent. The sites themselves are surrounded by fairly dense forest. Sites 3 and 4 are in a small, grassy field that separates the parking area from the state-forest road. These sites are wide open and quite spacious but not very private. They are also close to the pit toilets, which are the only facilities at this primitive campground. Even though sites 3 and 4 are right off the small parking area, they can still offer seclusion, especially since there won't be any road traffic later in the evening.

Site 6 is also a very spacious site just to the left of the restrooms. If you're going to camp closer to the road, though (that is, if you couldn't score a pond site), choose site 5. You'll have a very short lug-in from the parking area, which gives this site a pleasant, isolated feel. It's also set within a dense grove of mixed deciduous and coniferous trees that shield it from the state forest road.

Site 7 is a roomy and private site off to the left as you start to wind down the short road that leads to the pond sites. It's also right across from the water fountain. The dense wall of woods surrounding the site gives it a wilderness feel.

> *Whether you're into hiking, biking, paddling, or horseback riding, you won't run out of things to do at Beartown State Forest.*

RATINGS

Beauty: ☆☆☆☆☆
Privacy: ☆☆☆☆
Spaciousness: ☆☆☆
Quiet: ☆☆☆☆☆
Security: ☆☆☆☆
Cleanliness: ☆☆☆☆

KEY INFORMATION

All sites have at least one picnic table and a fire ring. From sites 8 and 12, you'll have easy access to the footpath leading to the shore of Benedict Pond. Site 8 is more open than the other sites in the pondside neighborhood. Like site 12, it's near but not directly on the pond.

From site 12, you'll still have a good pond view from your table, but you probably won't see the water through your tent's front flaps. Site 12 is also on a small rise, which gives it good drainage and makes it a better vantage point. Sites 9 through 11 are situated right along the edge of the pond. Site 11 is the choice pond spot. This really is a perfect, dramatically sculpted site. It sits on a small rise that looks out onto the placid waters of Benedict Pond and the rolling hills that frame the water. The pond-access trail runs by the right side of the site, but that's no bother. Besides offering a view filled with dramatic scenery, the site is well isolated. With its pond-facing orientation and the ring of wildflowers and maples surrounding it, this site offers the best of both the pond and the woods.

Since you're bound to spend lots of time just sitting and drinking in the view (and who knows, you may make some new friends happy to share the experience), know that there are two picnic tables at this site. You could take this site for a week and never have to leave once. You can paddle, swim, and fish right from your campsite. Even doing nothing in a site like this is spectacular.

Sites 9 and 10 have equally dramatic locations next to the pond. The two individually are a bit smaller than site 11, and they're a bit close together, but this would be a perfect pair for a group, and you couldn't ask for two more-scenic spots. All in all, sites 9, 10, and 11 are classic pondside campsites. It's worth planning way ahead for a few nights in one of these sites.

The campground is very quiet, even during the day. The only sounds you'll hear are the woodland birds talking back and forth, the soft splash of a canoe or kayak paddle out in the pond, and perhaps the whiz of a line being cast into the water.

With all this solitude, there's still plenty to do within Beartown State Forest. There's even a larger beach and day-use area up the state-forest road before you get to the campground. To hit the hiking trails right from the campground, follow Benedict Pond Road (the paved road

MAP

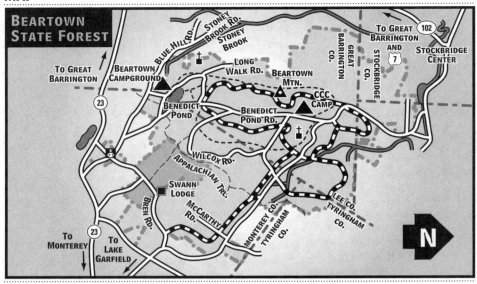

running through the forest and past the campground) to the Wildcat, Turkey, Sky Peak, and Airplane trails. I've never cycled it before, but I've heard from mountain-biking buddies in this neck of the woods that the Airplane Trail is one you won't want to miss.

All the above trails are multiuse trails, so you'll see hikers and bikers. Be careful, be aware, and share the trails. Horses are allowed on these trails as well, but you might not see many, since there is a separate bridle trail. The blue-blazed trails are the hiking trails, the red-blazed trail is the bridle trail, and the white blazes indicate the Appalachian Trail. The orange-blazed trails are open to everyone—hikers, bikers, horses, and off-road vehicles.

Note: *Shortly before press time, the Massachusetts Department of Conservation and Recreation announced that the campground and Benedict Pond will be closed until about July 30, 2012, while the dam on the pond is repaired. In addition, a number of park enhancements will be implemented, including installation of an accessible trail and bridge from the lower campsites to the beach, accessible picnic areas, new cooking facilities, and improved campsite access. For more information, visit* **mass.gov/dcr/parks/western/bear.htm.**

GETTING THERE

From US 7 in Great Barrington, take MA 23 east 5.3 miles to Monterey. Turn left onto Blue Hill Road and follow the brown lead-in signs 2.2 miles to the park entrance on the right (Benedict Pond Road).

GPS COORDINATES

N42° 12.150879'
W73° 17.339122'

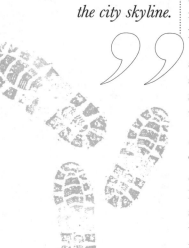

> *The Boston Harbor Islands offer a unique combination of wilderness island camping set against the backdrop of the city skyline.*

IT'S A BIT SURREAL to be camping on an island and sitting on a rocky ocean beach with a view of the Boston skyline. The soundtrack includes the soft crackle of the campfire, the birds and other sounds of the forest . . . and planes coming in and out of Logan International Airport. After all, you're just minutes from the city.

Make no mistake, though: this is primitive island camping. Even though you'll probably take a ferry to get here and you can see the city skyline in the distance, you must be 100 percent self-sufficient. Bring all your food, all your water, anything you need to cook with—*everything*.

Camping on Grape, Bumpkin, or Lovells Island is a true island-camping experience (Peddocks Island will also offer camping beginning in the summer of 2012). Staying here will necessitate a little extra planning, but the payoff is well worth it.

GRAPE ISLAND

The order in which these are presented is roughly my order of preference: Grape Island, Bumpkin Island, and Lovells Island. On Grape Island, the individual and group sites are spread out along a delightful maze of trails that wind through low scrub brush, wild berries, and a mixed forest of mostly sumac, birch, and pine.

Benches and picnic tables are arranged at strategic spots along the hiking trails. The ocean breezes and views of Boston Harbor and the city skyline are well worth stopping for a moment or two. While Bostonians are sweltering in the city, you'll be nice and cool out on the water. Once the sun dips below the horizon, you may even be tempted to pull on a fleece.

When camping on Grape Island, be sure to explore all the trails. It's a fairly small island, so it won't really take long. The entire island is filled with spectacularly scenic spots. One trail drops you right down on a rocky beach. Swimming is allowed here, but it's at your own risk.

RATINGS

Beauty: ☆☆☆☆☆
Privacy: ☆☆☆☆☆
Spaciousness: ☆☆☆
Quiet: ☆☆☆☆
Security: ☆☆☆☆
Cleanliness: ☆☆☆☆

Head off to the right as you come onto the island from the dock. Then turn left at your first opportunity—that trail leads up to the individual sites. The sites here aren't huge, but since you're arriving carrying only what you could bring with you on the boat, that shouldn't pose too much of a problem. Check in with the ranger before proceeding to the sites (especially since they're not all that well marked), and make sure you've brought along your camping permit.

The first site you'll come to, on the right, is very open and sunny. Across from site 1 on the left is site 2, which is completely shaded by the low, dense forest. Overall, the sites on the left side of the trail will feel much cooler on those really still, muggy summer days.

Site 3 is tucked way in on the right. It's behind the composting toilet, though. You might not want to be too close to that—especially when the wind is right. Site 4, on the left, is another densely shaded site.

Both sites 5 and 6 are bright, sunny ones, but they're also sheltered from the trail by the forest. Site 7 is also nicely shaded. Site 8 is tucked off to the left and shaded by a grove of young birch trees. Site 9 is another that is partly sunny and partly shaded. Off to the left, it's also sheltered from the trail. Site 10 is well off the hiking trail to the right. This one is also both sunny and shaded. It's set farther back off the trail than are the other sites. The trails that wind through the sites and around the island have a nice, soft, grassy surface.

The group camping sites aren't the big fields you find at inland campgrounds. Rather, they're more like a series of nooks and crannies set off the trail. The group sites are to the left when you arrive on the island. Like the individual sites, they aren't well marked, so check with the ranger if you have any questions. Camping is by reservation only, so it's unlikely that anyone will steal your site.

The first section of site 1 has a tent platform. A small part of the site is tucked in beneath a tree. Another section of the site, across the trail, has a bit more room than the first two parts and is set a bit farther back from the trail. Still another spacious part of the site is set beneath a canopy of trees.

KEY INFORMATION

ADDRESS:	408 Atlantic Ave., Suite 225 Boston MA 02110
OPERATED BY:	Massachusetts Department of Conservation and Recreation
INFORMATION:	617-223-8666
OPEN:	Mid-June– Labor Day
SITES:	26 individual sites and 4 group sites on 3 islands (Peddocks Island will also offer camping beginning in summer 2012)
EACH SITE:	Picnic table; some have grills
ASSIGNMENT:	By reservation only: 877-422-6762, reserve america.com
REGISTRATION:	Check in with ranger on island; camping permit required
FACILITIES:	Composting toilets
PARKING:	Park at or near ferry terminals; call 617-223-8666 for ferry schedules
FEE:	Massachusetts residents, $6; nonresidents, $8; group camping, $25
RESTRICTIONS:	*Pets:* Prohibited *Fires:* Campfires permitted below high-tide line *Alcohol:* Prohibited *Vehicles:* Prohibited *Other:* Pack-in, pack-out policy; 2-week maximum stay; no water or food available

While you're on Grape Island, explore the ruins of a 19th-century foundation near the dock. The house was occupied by Amos Pendleton, described as "an old hermit with a dangerous temper."

BUMPKIN ISLAND

Bumpkin Island definitely has steeper hills and trails than does Grape—it's a bit easier to navigate in terms of where you're going to find the campsites, though. The low forest and ground cover are also much denser on Bumpkin than on Grape. Most of the campsites are situated along a side trail that extends from the main trail that bisects the island. This main trail was actually paved at one point, as Bumpkin was host to first a children's hospital and then a military training ground.

To the left, site 1 tucked is back off the trail. It's partially shaded and fairly good-sized compared with some of the others. Site 2, also to the left, is much smaller. It's a bit open to the trails leading to sites 4 and 3. Site 4, on the right, is also open to the trail. Both sites are partially shaded by the low, dense forest.

Site 3 wraps around, so it's a bit more secluded. Site 4 is open to the trail and next to another trail leading into site 3. Site 5 is nicely shaded; it's down from the trail to the left. Site 6, off to the right, is a nice open site next to a sprawling sumac tree. Across the trail is site 7, which is shadier and slightly smaller.

On the right side of the trail is site 8, which is small, circular, and very sunny despite being ringed by dense walls of forest. Site 9 is off to the left from a small clearing in the trail. It's set against a couple of good-sized sumac trees. Site 10, the most secluded of the bunch, lies off to the left of the trail that leads you past all the campsites. This is a larger site as well, surrounded by dense shrub and forest yet also sunny and open to the sky.

Group site 1 would be a good-sized site at a mainland campground. It's open to the sky and ringed by a wall of short sumac, with one defiant clump growing off to the side within the site. Across the trail is the historic site of the Burrage Children's Hospital, which was once a place for crippled youngsters to spend the summer. Group site 2 is well off the central trail and very secluded. It's about the same size as group site 1. There's also big open field designated as a picnic area down on the western side of Bumpkin.

Both Grape's and Bumpkin's individual sites lie along a relatively short section of trail. I like the character and seclusion of the Grape sites a bit better, however. Both islands could benefit from marking the path to the sites better, but both are also fairly small islands, so you can't go too far wrong.

LOVELLS ISLAND

Bumpkin and Grape islands are in Hingham Bay, so they're a bit more protected. But Lovells Island is well out in Boston Harbor, so it gets a bit more noise from marine traffic and Logan Airport. You can hear all that from any of the Boston Harbor Islands, but you're a lot closer when you're on Lovells. Still, the size and historic aspects of Lovells, and the dramatic cliffs off the northeastern side of the island, make it well worth checking out. Once you start exploring, you'll easily be able to tune out the sounds of the city.

From the dock, you'll follow a well-worn path of old pavement. I'd wager those paths were paved during World War II, when Lovells was used for coastal gun emplacements. When you reach a fork in the road, the left path will appear to follow the shore of the island, while the right path goes up a small hill toward the fort. The campsites are off the left path. Like the paths at Grape and Bumpkin, this one could benefit from being better marked.

Site 1 is on the low road, to the right. It's partially shaded and set back and down from the road, so it offers a nice sense of seclusion. Site 2 is also down off the road. Follow a short footpath just past site 1 to reach it. This nicely shaded site is covered by loosely spaced sumac. Most of these sites have a fire ring, grill, and picnic table.

Site 3 is also off to the right, connected to site 2 by a short footpath. This is a pretty cozy site, but it's very open to the sun and sky. Site 4, tucked well off the road, has a tent platform and grill, and it's fairly close to the composting toilet. That may be good for some, not so good for others.

Site 5 must be one of the group sites, as it's quite large. Very spacious and open, it's on the other side of the composting toilet from site 4. It's also conjoined with what appears to be another site with a picnic table and grill. Site 6, a nicely shaded offshoot, is set off from the open space of site 5. One more site on the right side of the road, down near the end, is nicely secluded and close to the beach. It's on the small side, but its location is perfect.

A couple of sites appear to be unused. The DCR is rightfully very careful about island conservation, so site placements and numbers probably change here more frequently than on the mainland. This fact, along with the virtually nonexistent site markings, means you should not only check with the DCR when making your reservation to get exactly the site you're looking for, you should check with the ranger on the island to make sure the site you occupy is indeed the site you intended.

MAP

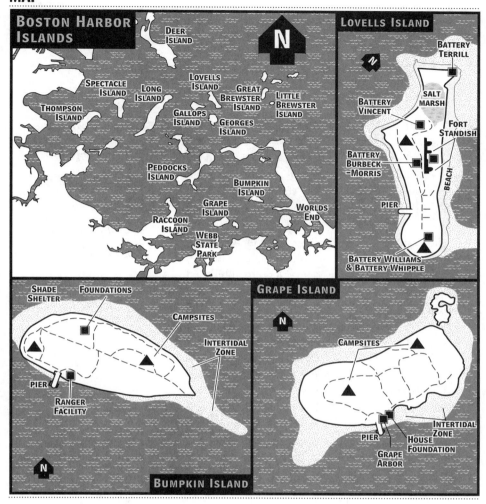

GETTING THERE

Take the ferry from either the Marriott Long Wharf hotel in Boston or from Quincy Harbor. The ferries run interisland loops. Take the south loop from Quincy Harbor for Grape and Bumpkin, and the north loop from Boston or George's Island for Lovells. Call 617-223-8666 for ferry information and trip planning.

GPS COORDINATES

GRAPE ISLAND
N42° 16.098661'
W70° 55.231755'

LOVELLS ISLAND
N42° 19.605460'
W70° 55.578811'

BUMPKIN ISLAND
N42° 16.852992'
W70° 53.944774'

44
CLARKSBURG
STATE PARK

CLARKSBURG **S**TATE **P**ARK is up in the northwestern corner of Massachusetts, along the Vermont border. The sites at the park's moderately sized campground are carved out of a dense forest of pine, spruce, and hemlock that gives the woods a dark, cool feeling. Even on the most brilliant, sunny days, the whole campground is immersed in the shade of the verdant forest.

The coniferous trees blanket most of the campground with a velvety layer of pine needles. The sites are spread out along a large, central loop road bisected by a crossroad. Sites 9 through 14 (including site 12A) are situated along the crossroad; the rest are on the outer loops.

You can reserve most of the sites. Sites 1, 4, 10, 11, 12, 14, 18, 23, 25, and 29 are the first-come, first-served sites. Those along the inner side of the campground loop and the crossroad have the most densely forested feel. The sites facing Mauserts Pond, although they are still quite a ways back from the water's edge and carved out of the forest, afford a bit more light through the trees and occasional glimpses of the pond.

Sites 1 and 2 are very spacious and have an isolated feeling. Even though the woods here are thick, you can catch a glimpse of Mauserts Pond from site 2. Sites 6 and 7 are pleasant and set down from the road, which adds to their privacy. Sites 10 and 11 are smaller than most of the other sites at Clarksburg State Park, and they're close to the facilities.

Along the stretch of the campground loop where you'll find sites 16 through 23, the sites are large and isolated from each other and from the rest of the sites. These are all decent sites for tent camping, as you'll enjoy a sense of solitude here. More hardwoods are mixed into the forest along this portion of the campground loop road. The brilliant-green leaves of the maples in summer brighten the scenery.

> *The campground at Clarksburg State Park has a dark, cool, sylvan air even on the most brilliant summer days.*

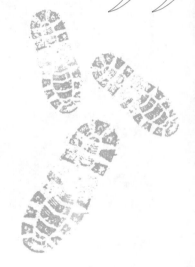

RATINGS

Beauty: ☆ ☆ ☆ ☆
Privacy: ☆ ☆ ☆
Spaciousness: ☆ ☆ ☆ ☆
Quiet: ☆ ☆ ☆ ☆
Security: ☆ ☆ ☆ ☆
Cleanliness: ☆ ☆ ☆ ☆

KEY INFORMATION

ADDRESS: 1199 Middle Rd. Clarksburg, MA 01247

OPERATED BY: Massachusetts Department of Conservation and Recreation

INFORMATION: 413-664-8345 (summer), 413-663-8469 (mid-Oct.–mid-April)

OPEN: Late May–early Sept.

SITES: 45 (including 3 that are sometimes set aside for camp hosts)

EACH SITE: Fire ring, picnic table

ASSIGNMENT: First-come, first-served or by reservation: 877-422-6762, reserve america.com

REGISTRATION: At ranger station

FACILITIES: Flush toilets, beach area, boat launch

PARKING: At sites

FEE: Massachusetts residents, $12; nonresidents, $14

RESTRICTIONS: *Pets:* Dogs on leash only
Fires: Fire rings only
Alcohol: Prohibited
Vehicles: Maximum 2 per site
Other: Reservations require 2-night minimum stay; campground office hours 8 a.m.–7 p.m.; 14-day maximum stay

Moving farther along the one-way campground loop road, you'll come to site 23, which is tremendous. Set way back from the road, it's rather large and has a calming sense of wilderness seclusion. The forest directly overhead is clear, so you'll also get light filtering down and glimpses of the night sky (once you've put your campfire out and your eyes adjust to the dark). The only issue is that it's occasionally set aside for campground management, as are sites 22 and 29.

Sites 25 and above are a bit smaller than most of the others, particularly the sites situated along the outside of the campground loop road, but they are still attractive and offer a private atmosphere, as they're set within the dense coniferous forest. The walls of pine and spruce here form an effective barrier between the individual sites. Site 29 is the exception, but this is a large site well suited for a group or family.

Site 31 sits within its own clearing. This is a good spot if you have smaller kids, as you'll find it easier to keep an eye on them. Site 33 looks much the same but is a bit smaller.

It seems that site 36 has vanished from the Clarksburg State Park campground loop. In its place is a trailhead that leads off in the direction of the Mauserts Loop Trail. Perhaps the site was sacrificed to make a spot for the trailhead—not a bad tradeoff, if you ask me.

Finishing up the campground loop road, sites 35 through 44 are smaller than some of the other isolated, larger sites and those along the outer loop. However, thanks to the deep, dense nature of Clarksburg's forest, they still provide privacy and isolation.

Overall, the sensation here is one of being sequestered in a thick forest. There's a hush over the place even during daylight hours. In the evening, all you're likely to hear is the snap and crackle of campfires.

During the day, you'll definitely want to check out Mauserts Pond. A footpath leads to the pond right across from site 25. If you bring a canoe or kayak, it might be easier to head over to the day-use area, which has a boat launch and beach.

Several fairly lengthy hiking trails wind through Clarksburg State Park. The Mauserts Loop Trail leads from the campground and crosses Beaver Creek, then

MAP

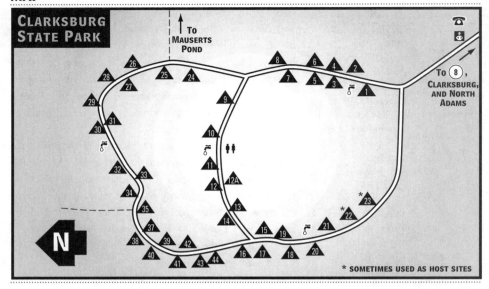

CLARKSBURG STATE PARK

To MAUSERTS POND

To (8), CLARKSBURG, AND NORTH ADAMS

N

* SOMETIMES USED AS HOST SITES

brings you up toward Vermont. The Horrigan Road Trail veers west about two-thirds of the way to the Vermont border, after which the trail is called (appropriately enough) the Vermont Line Trail. The Bog Trail curves around the northern end of the pond and brings you to the beach and boathouse.

GETTING THERE

Follow MA 8 through Clarksburg heading toward Vermont until you see the signs for Clarksburg State Park, on the left.

GPS COORDINATES

N42° 44.029641'
W73° 4.571056'

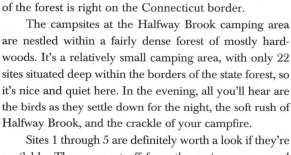

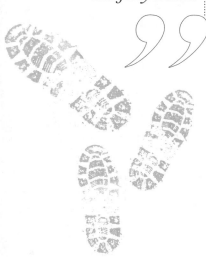

When you're camping at Granville State Forest, you'll fall asleep to the sounds of the forest and the soft whisper of Halfway Brook.

YOU'LL FIND **GRANVILLE STATE FOREST** in the southwestern corner of Massachusetts. The southern edge of the forest is right on the Connecticut border.

The campsites at the Halfway Brook camping area are nestled within a fairly dense forest of mostly hardwoods. It's a relatively small camping area, with only 22 sites situated deep within the borders of the state forest, so it's nice and quiet here. In the evening, all you'll hear are the birds as they settle down for the night, the soft rush of Halfway Brook, and the crackle of your campfire.

Sites 1 through 5 are definitely worth a look if they're available. These are set off from the main campground and face West Hartland Road. Site 1 couldn't be any closer to Halfway Brook, which makes this site particularly attractive. It sits right next to a small pond formed by the intersection of Halfway and Small brooks. Sites 1 and 2 are very private, as there is plenty of forest between them and the rest of the campground. Adding to the sense of seclusion, sites 1 and 2 are set farther back off the road. Any other sounds you might hear from the rest of the campground are obscured by the light whisper of Halfway Brook tumbling by in the background.

Sites 3, 4, and 5 are also nicely isolated but a bit closer to the rest of the campsites in the main loop. The rear border of these sites abuts the borders of sites 6, 8, and 9 in the main campground loop. These sites are set within more open forest, so they're spacious but a bit less private—even though they're still accessed via West Hartland Road and not via the campground loop. Parking for sites 1 through 5 is also separate from the rest of the campground.

Adjacent sites 6 and 7 are very large. There's a fair degree of privacy between these sites and the rest of the campground, but the forest is loosely spaced between them. This would be a good pair of sites for a larger group. Site 8 is nicely isolated, nestled into the forest right where

RATINGS

Beauty: ✩ ✩ ✩ ✩
Privacy: ✩ ✩ ✩ ✩
Spaciousness: ✩ ✩ ✩ ✩ ✩
Quiet: ✩ ✩ ✩ ✩
Security: ✩ ✩ ✩ ✩
Cleanliness: ✩ ✩ ✩ ✩

you turn off the campground road to the parking area. It's surrounded by fairly dense forest, so it offers a strong sense of seclusion from the rest of the campground.

The rest of the sites provide a blend of seclusion, spaciousness, and privacy, as they are set amid the dense mixed forest that shelters the campground. Site 11 is quite secluded. You make a short drive down to the site off the primary parking area in the center of the campground. Site 10 is close to the gently murmuring Halfway Brook.

Sites 12 and 14 are very spacious. Sites 19, 20, and 21 are all fairly close to each other and are a bit more open than some of the other sites. Sites 15 and 19 are near a small, grassy field, out behind the restrooms. Sites 13 and 21, right on the campground loop road, are a bit too open for my taste.

An elaborate network of hiking trails winds through the rest of the forest. Across the street from the campground are trailheads for the Ordway Trail and the Civilian Conservation Corps (CCC) Trail. From the CCC Trail, you can loop around on the Corduroy Trail, which heads out past the forest headquarters and travels through a wetland before reconnecting with the CCC Trail. The hiking trails on this side of West Hartland Road are fairly flat.

On the same side of the road as the campground are the Halfway Brook Trail and the Hubbard River Trail, which leads down to where the Hubbard River Campground used to be. You can also access the Woods Trail, which travels up and over a small ridgeline, and the Ore Hill Trail, which follows the eastern border of the forest. The trails on this side of the road travel either along or up and over Ore Hill. The aforementioned trails are all multiuse trails, so you can hike, mountain-bike, and ride horses. Keeping this in mind, exercise appropriate caution and courtesy. Even though you might feel you're out in the middle of nowhere at Granville State Forest, you may find that's just the sensation you were seeking.

KEY INFORMATION

ADDRESS:	323 W. Hartland Rd. Granville, MA 01034
OPERATED BY:	Massachusetts Department of Conservation and Recreation
INFORMATION:	413-357-6611
OPEN:	Late May– early Sept.
SITES:	20
EACH SITE:	Fire ring, picnic table
ASSIGNMENT:	First-come, first-served or by reservation (recommended): 877-422-6762, reserveamerica.com
REGISTRATION:	At ranger station
FACILITIES:	Flush toilets, hot showers, phone
PARKING:	At sites or in central parking area
FEE:	Massachusetts residents, $12; non-residents, $14
RESTRICTIONS:	*Pets:* On leash only *Fires:* In fire rings *Alcohol:* Prohibited *Vehicles:* Maximum 2 per site; no ORVs *Other:* Reservations require 2-night minimum stay; office hours 8 a.m.– 10 p.m.; quiet hours 10 p.m.–7 a.m; 14-day maximum stay; Hubbard River area remains closed until further notice

MAP

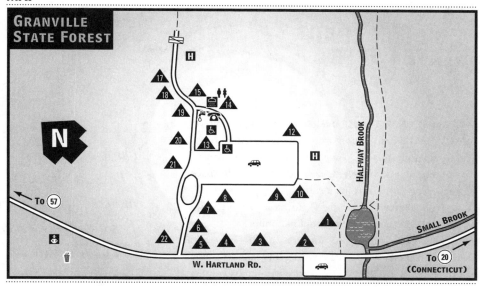

GETTING THERE

From the intersection of MA 8 and MA 57 in New Boston, follow MA 57 west to West Hartland Road. Head south on West Hartland Road until you see signs for the forest and the campground.

GPS COORDINATES

N42° 3.580413'
W72° 58.280439'

46

MOHAWK TRAIL STATE FOREST

A SENSE OF REVERENCE OVERCOMES you upon entering Mohawk Trail State Forest. The woods here have a cathedralesque quality. Take a moment as you drive in to get out of your vehicle. Gaze at the tall, nicely spaced spruce–pine forest forming a canopy over you, and relish the "wise silence of the forest" (to quote Ralph Waldo Emerson) and the delightful scent of conifer.

This is an older-growth forest, as the trees are all at least 100 feet tall, with some considerably taller than that. At the forest floor, the tree trunks are quite massive; there isn't much in the way of an understory, so the forest has an open feel to it. The sunlight filters down through the giant conifers in broken shafts, and most breezes are captured by the long arms of the trees. Parts of the forest are also interspersed with maple, birch, and other hardy deciduous trees and the offspring of the giant evergreens.

The sites in the first cluster are set close together but remain fairly open for such a densely forested area. These sites are clean and spacious, but not quite as private as you might expect when you first see the forest.

In the loop with sites 36 through 56 down near the Cold River, you hear the sounds of the forest birds and the rushing water. The sites right along the river are the best—they're set within a beautiful, loose grove of mixed hardwoods and conifers. RVs are allowed in Mohawk Trail State Forest, but you won't find any in this part of the campground, primarily because they're unable to negotiate the extremely tight turn at the end of the road.

The riverside sites are spectacular. They are a bit open to each other but set near the Cold River. Sites 45 through 48 all sit right on the riverbanks at the end of the loop, so they're even more isolated than the other sites in this cluster. Sites 46 and 47 are the perfect riverside spots. Across the river from site 47 is the Mohawk State Forest picnic area, but the day-trippers will be gone by the time you're lighting your campfire to cook dinner.

> *The towering forest at this campground's entrance is breathtaking. If that doesn't get you, wait until you see the campsites along Cold River.*

RATINGS

Beauty: ☆☆☆☆☆
Privacy: ☆☆☆☆
Spaciousness: ☆☆☆☆
Quiet: ☆☆☆☆☆
Security: ☆☆☆☆
Cleanliness: ☆☆☆☆☆

KEY INFORMATION

ADDRESS: P.O. Box 7/MA 2
Charlemont, MA
01339
OPERATED BY: Massachusetts
Department of
Conservation and
Recreation
INFORMATION: 413-339-5504
OPEN: Early May–
mid-Oct.
SITES: 49 sites, 6 cabins
(available year-
round), 4 group
sites
EACH SITE: Fire ring,
picnic table
ASSIGNMENT: First-come, first-
served or by
reservation (rec-
ommended):
877-422-6762,
reserveamerica.com
REGISTRATION: At ranger station
FACILITIES: Flush toilets, water
spigots, showers,
handicap-accessible
restrooms
PARKING: At sites
FEE: Massachusetts
residents, $12;
nonresidents, $14;
$25 for group site;
$30–$50 for cabins
RESTRICTIONS: *Pets:* Dogs on
leash only
Fires: In fire rings
only
Alcohol: Prohibited
Vehicles: Parking at
sites only
Other: Reservations
require 2-night
minimum stay;
campground office
hours 8 a.m.–10
p.m.; quiet hours
10 p.m.–7 a.m.; 14-
day maximum stay

The sites numbered in the 30s are spacious but are also exposed and set on a hard dirt surface. Sites 14 through 22 sit off a short road that leaves the upper campground loop. Sites 15 and 16 are small but sweet riverside sites on the riverbanks, a bit higher than the sites in the 40s and 50s. Site 22, at the end of this small loop, is the key site in this cluster—very spacious and private.

The whole 14-through-22 loop is set in a grove of enormous spruce trees, so you get plenty of shade and that earthy, deep-woods scent. And of course, the Cold River rushes right by the campsites, so all your senses are satisfied.

The main section of the campground with sites 2 through 8 and 23 through 33 is decent, but the sites offer minimal privacy. A developed forest canopy gives this area a lot of shade, but the minimal undergrowth doesn't make for much seclusion.

When you come to camp at Mohawk Trail State Forest, look for the sites in the upper 40s and lower 50s at the end of the campground and near the Cold River. Those are where you'll want to be. If that doesn't work, go for the 14-through-22 loop.

Remember: This is black-bear country, so all the appropriate precautions apply to food, garbage, and even clothes upon which you may have spilled food. When you're turning in for the night, hide anything that may retain food scents safely in your car.

MAP

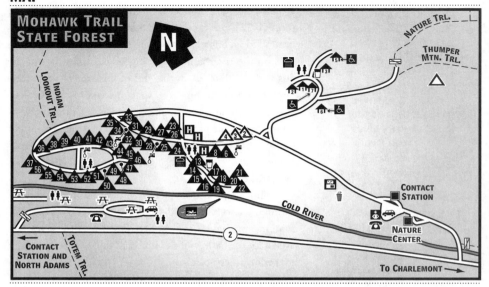

GETTING THERE

Follow MA 2 east from
North Adams until you see
the signs for Mohawk Trail
State Forest, on the left.

GPS COORDINATES

N42° 38.192096'
W72° 56.139879'

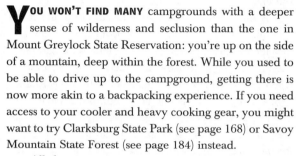

47
MOUNT GREYLOCK CAMPGROUND

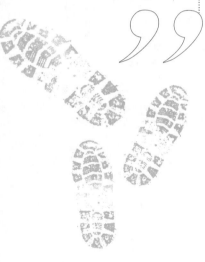

Here you'll be deep in the woods, perched on the mountainside, and in the midst of a massive network of hiking and biking trails.

YOU WON'T FIND MANY campgrounds with a deeper sense of wilderness and seclusion than the one in Mount Greylock State Reservation: you're up on the side of a mountain, deep within the forest. While you used to be able to drive up to the campground, getting there is now more akin to a backpacking experience. If you need access to your cooler and heavy cooking gear, you might want to try Clarksburg State Park (see page 168) or Savoy Mountain State Forest (see page 184) instead.

All these sites are remote, private, and spread out. Some of them are a bit small, but their rustic charm and deep-wilderness seclusion are irresistible. The sites are situated along the main campground road. Each is nestled within the dense forest of mixed deciduous and coniferous trees.

The 15 individual tent sites lie off either side of the main trail leading through the campground. Coming up the Hopper Trail, you'll turn right into the campground toward the 15 tent sites, the campground pavilion, and the outhouses. Following that path through the campground past all the tent sites will bring you to the Stony Ledge Group Area and one of the lean-to sites.

Turn left off the Hopper Trail to get to the Balsam, Spruce, and Chimney group sites and one of the lean-tos. Heading south off the campground road from the Hopper Road Trail or just in front of the Balsam group site will bring you to the Birch and Cherry group sites, as well as the Lower Group Area and another of the lean-to sites.

The forest is a dense mix of hardwoods and conifers, young and old, so the variety of the forest is visually stunning. After the sun goes down, the thick forest reflects the light from your campfire, making the trees look like a wall surrounding your site.

And again, this is semideveloped backpacking, not car camping. If you can't carry it in—or, just as importantly,

RATINGS

Beauty: ✿ ✿ ✿ ✿ ✿
Privacy: ✿ ✿ ✿ ✿
Spaciousness: ✿ ✿ ✿ ✿
Quiet: ✿ ✿ ✿ ✿ ✿
Security: ✿ ✿ ✿ ✿ ✿
Cleanliness: ✿ ✿ ✿ ✿

carry it out—try one of the other nearby campgrounds like Clarksburg, Savoy Mountain, or Mohawk Trail.

You'll find plenty to do here during the day. Camped right on the side of Mount Greylock, you're in the midst of a giant network of trails for hiking and mountain biking. The Appalachian Trail cuts through here, so you may run into some thru-hikers on and around Greylock.

A number of trailheads lead right out of the campground. The Hopper Trail leads from the parking area through the campground and continues to the summit of Mount Greylock. Just beyond the footbridge, past the Birch and Cherry group areas, you'll find the Roaring Brook Trail, the Deer Hill Trail, and the Circular Trail. The March Cataract Trail, near the Chimney Group Site, leads to some dramatic waterfalls. On the other side of the mountain is the classic Thunderbolt Trail, one of New England's earliest ski trails, cut by the Civilian Conservation Corps. I've descended the mighty Thunderbolt only once, and I have somewhat-fond memories of the trail. It was in the late winter, so I brought out my telemark skis for the occasion. It was downright ugly—the dense late-winter snow grabbed my skis and refused to let go. The mountain won that day, but I had a blast nevertheless.

KEY INFORMATION

ADDRESS:	P.O. Box 138 Lanesborough, MA 01237
OPERATED BY:	Massachusetts Department of Conservation and Recreation
INFORMATION:	413-499-4262
OPEN:	Year-round (off-season is first-come, first-served)
SITES:	15 sites, 7 group sites, 3 lean-to sites
EACH SITE:	Fire ring or stone hearth, picnic table
ASSIGNMENT:	Reservations required Memorial Day–Columbus Day; lean-tos first-come, first-served
REGISTRATION:	At ranger station
FACILITIES:	Pit toilets
PARKING:	At Hopper Road trailhead (a 2.5-mile hike to campground) or Rockwell Road (a 1.3-mile hike)
FEE:	Massachusetts residents, $6; nonresidents, $8; group camping, $25
RESTRICTIONS:	*Pets:* On leash only *Fires:* In fire rings only *Alcohol:* Prohibited *Vehicles:* Parking at Hopper Road trailhead year-round, at Rockwell Road late May–early Nov. *Other:* Reservations require 1-night minimum stay; 4-person maximum per tent site, 12-person maximum per group site

MAP

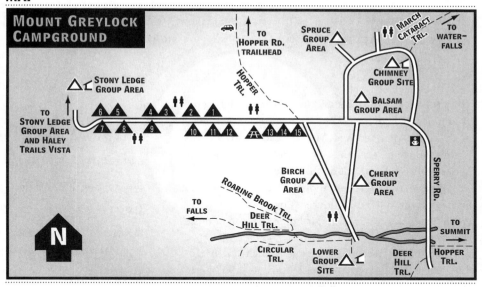

GETTING THERE

Follow US 7 and MA 20 north through Lanesborough, then follow signs to the Mount Greylock State Reservation headquarters. The campground is on Sperry Road, which is several miles up the auto road heading toward the summit.

GPS COORDINATES

N42° 38.050883'
W73° 11.376693'

48
NICKERSON STATE PARK

IT'S NO SECRET THAT **CAPE COD** gets packed during the summer. Just look at MA 3 leading toward the Sagamore Bridge or I-495 and MA 25 leading toward the Bourne Bridge on a summer Friday night, and you'll see lines of cars waiting to get on the Cape.

What may be a secret, though, is that you can still find some solitude and wilderness on the Cape. Nickerson State Park, in Brewster, is home to some of those rare, remote spots.

Part of the reason Nickerson is such an incredible refuge is its size: it's huge. Within its 1,955 acres and among its 418 campsites, you can find all sorts of places to quietly lose yourself in the rolling pine forests that blanket the park. This is one of the most densely forested areas on the Cape. The forest itself is beautiful, with loosely spaced balsams, firs, and pines. Once you've decided on a spot to pitch your tent, take a quiet moment for a deep breath. When there's an onshore breeze, you can smell the earthy scent of the coniferous forest and the salty tang of the nearby ocean in the same breath.

There aren't any sites within Nickerson specifically set aside for tent campers, but several of the eight discrete areas lend themselves particularly well to tents. Look for sites in areas 2, 3, 5, or 7. Areas 2 and 3 are about a mile from the main entrance and are in open loops. Each area has its own restroom along with several drinking-water spigots.

Area 5 is about 0.5 mile from the entrance on the way to Flax Pond. Several of the sites here are open and loosely spaced, especially 12, 14, and 16 through 18. A few pathways lead off the bluff down to Flax Pond, where you can swim, fish, paddle, or just enjoy a few moments walking along the water.

Area 7 has a number of loosely spaced sites. Of the 46 sites in this area, the 27-through-29 and

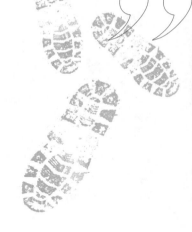

> *Nickerson State Park is quite large, but it's also one of the few spots on the Cape where you can find a slice of wilderness for yourself, even during the busy summer season.*

RATINGS

Beauty: ☆ ☆ ☆ ☆
Privacy: ☆ ☆ ☆
Spaciousness: ☆ ☆ ☆
Quiet: ☆ ☆ ☆ ☆
Security: ☆ ☆ ☆ ☆
Cleanliness: ☆ ☆ ☆ ☆

ADDRESS: 3488 Main St.
MA 6A
Brewster, MA
02631-1521

OPERATED BY: Massachusetts
Department of
Conservation and
Recreation

INFORMATION: 508-896-3491

OPEN: Early May–late Oct.

SITES: 406 throughout
8 areas; 9 group
sites, 6 yurts

EACH SITE: Fire ring,
picnic table

ASSIGNMENT: First-come, first-
served; reserva-
tions strongly
recommended:
877-422-6762,
reserveamerica.com

REGISTRATION: At main entrance
on MA 6A Mon.–
Fri., 9 a.m.–3 p.m.,
or call 508-896-4615

FACILITIES: Restrooms, hot
showers, pay
phone

PARKING: At sites and day-
use areas

FEE: Massachusetts
residents, $15,
nonresidents, $17;
$25 for group site;
$30–$40 for yurts

RESTRICTIONS: *Pets:* On leash only
Fires: In fire rings
only; do not leave
unattended
Alcohol: Not allowed
Vehicles: At sites
only
Other: Quiet hours
10 p.m.–7 a.m.;
14-day maximum
stay, 2-day
minimum stay

30-through-36 clusters are particularly isolated. These are great if you're with a group and can secure all the sites within a cluster. The sites in the low 30s are closest to Higgins Pond. Some of these sites, especially the ones nearest the water, have sandy areas, so if you have a set of those extra-large tent stakes for securing your nylon dome to loosely packed surfaces, be sure to bring them along.

Even if you take the last site in the park (which is not outside the realm of possibility if you come during July or August), you're still in for some sweet tent camping. Even on those sticky summer nights when the weather is hot and muggy, there are often cool breezes blowing through the forest and over the bluffs.

The several kettle ponds (glacial ponds fed by groundwater or precipitation) found throughout the park are among Nickerson's main attractions, especially for day-use visitors. Cliff Pond is the largest and the only pond in which waterskiing is allowed. Nevertheless, it still makes for beautiful paddling and swimming. Electric trolling motors are allowed in Flax Pond, if you want to drop a hook in the water in hopes that you'll find a hungry trout. The others—Higgins Pond, Eel Pond, Little Cliff Pond, Ruth Pond, Keeler's Pond, and Triangle Pond—are just for paddling, swimming, fishing, or pond-gazing.

You could spend days exploring the trails that wind through Nickerson before you crossed them all. You can hike, bike, and inline-skate (on the paved paths), and in the winter you can cross-country-ski and snowshoe. It's an amazing network of trails, and even on the busiest summer weekend you can still discover a little slice of wilderness solitude. Some of the trails end up in the park's neighbors' backyards, so if you find yourself on something that looks like private property, be respectful, turn around, and hike back into the park.

More than 8 miles of the 25-mile Cape Cod Rail Trail pass through the park, making it the perfect launch pad for cycling trips on the trail. You can pedal all the way to Dennis to the west of Nickerson State Park or to South Wellfleet to the east. Several businesses along the rail-trail rent bikes and helmets, if you didn't bring your own.

MAP

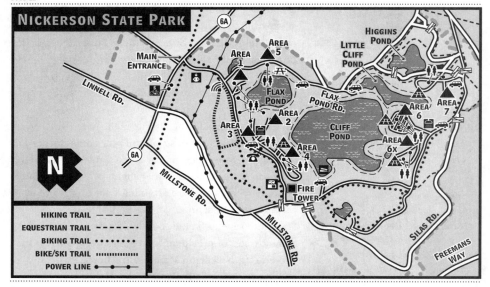

The Namskaket Sea Path also runs along the shoreline where Nickerson State Park faces Cape Cod Bay. It extends 2 miles from Linnell Landing in Brewster to Skaket Beach in Orleans. This is well worth exploring, especially at low tide, when you can walk across the mouth of Namskaket Creek. The sea path passes through an intertidal zone where you'll see seashells, hermit crabs, seabirds, and all sorts of seaweed and driftwood at the high-water mark.

While you're out there on the ocean side, take some time to explore the Brewster Flats. At low tide, it looks as if you could walk all the way to Provincetown at the end of the Cape. The flats are especially fun to experience with kids, who tend to notice things adults might otherwise pass by.

As peaceful as a stroll along the sandbars of the Brewster Flats can be, however, make sure that you pay attention and exercise caution. When the tide turns and starts coming in, it does so ferociously fast, rolling up and over the sandbars and advancing toward the shore with startling speed. I was caught out on the flats once

GETTING THERE
Follow US 6 East to MA 6A West. Follow MA 6A West for 1 mile or so to the entrance to the state park and campground, on your left.

GPS COORDINATES
N41° 46.533465'
W70° 1.843128'

in February—of all the times to be overtaken by the tide—and came back wet from the knees down.

Whether you spend most of your time at Nickerson State Park hiking the trails, biking along the rail-trail, relaxing by the shore of the ocean or by one of Nickerson's ponds, or just enjoying the last embers of your campfire, you'll discover a Cape Cod that isn't quite as crazy and crowded as you had imagined.

49
SAVOY MOUNTAIN
STATE FOREST

YOU COULD SEPARATE THE **45** campsites at Savoy Mountain State Forest by character into two very different groups. Most of the sites lie within the woods bordering the campground, but many are situated in a pastoral setting atop a hill covered by an open, grassy field punctuated by several large oaks, apple trees, and lilac bushes. This open, orchardlike field in the center of the campground affords a nice view of the sky. That unfettered view even extends to most of the sites set into the woods on the outer perimeter of the campground loop.

Sites 1 and 2 are tucked off on their own short road, which leads off to the right after you pass the ranger station at the campground entrance. These are the best sites in this part of the campground. They are spacious, isolated from each other and from the rest of the campground, and set in a grove of tall maple trees.

The forest framing the campground is a dense mix of mostly deciduous trees, so there's lots of shade and privacy. In these sites, light filters down to the forest floor in fractured shards.

The sites on the grassy hilltop at the center of the campground, including sites 34 to 45, are breezy, spacious, and open but not quite as private as the wooded sites. While I'm almost always a fan of more-secluded forested sites, many of these central sites have a fabulous pastoral feel about them: you'll feel as if you were camping in an orchard. The openness of these sites makes them perfect for some intense stargazing, or even sleeping under the stars. What sites 34 through 45 may lack in seclusion and privacy they more than make up for in their pastoral setting. Close by are large trees that break up the field, several bunches of brush, and wildflowers. This part of the campground would make a perfect setting for a remake of *The Sound of Music*.

On the outside of the campground loop road, sites 29 through 31 are set within the forest at the edge of the field.

> *Savoy Mountain State Forest has a fascinating blend of sites, some tucked into the woods, some on a grassy hill, and others nestled among apple trees.*

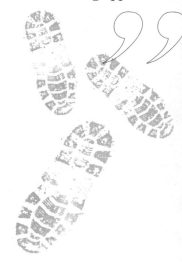

RATINGS

Beauty: ✪ ✪ ✪ ✪
Privacy: ✪ ✪ ✪ ✪
Spaciousness: ✪ ✪ ✪ ✪
Quiet: ✪ ✪ ✪ ✪ ✪
Security: ✪ ✪ ✪ ✪
Cleanliness: ✪ ✪ ✪ ✪

KEY INFORMATION

ADDRESS:	260 Central Shaft Rd. Florida, MA 01247
OPERATED BY:	Massachusetts Department of Conservation and Recreation
INFORMATION:	413-663-8469
OPEN:	Mid-May–mid-Oct.
SITES:	41 sites, 1 group site, 4 cabins (available year-round)
EACH SITE:	Fire ring, picnic table
ASSIGNMENT:	First-come, first-served; reservations recommended: 877-422-6762, reserveamerica .com
REGISTRATION:	At ranger station
FACILITIES:	Flush toilets, showers, water spigots
PARKING:	At sites
FEE:	Massachusetts residents, $12; non-residents, $14; $25 for group site; $30 for cabins
RESTRICTIONS:	*Pets:* On leash only *Fires:* In established fire rings only *Alcohol:* Not allowed *Vehicles:* Parking at sites only *Other:* Quiet hours 10 p.m.–7 a.m.; 14-day maximum stay and 2-day minimum stay for reservations

They share the benefits of the forest and the field, in that they're open but also feel somewhat secluded.

If these sites had nicknames, site 32 would be called the orchard site, as it is framed with several small apple trees. Site 31 would share that nickname, as it's also nicely isolated and has a couple of apple trees holding vigil at the entrance. If those are the orchard sites, then site 39 is the lilac site—it sits high on the open field, right next to a huge lilac bush.

Sites 8 through 21 are spaced out along the other side of the campground loop road. They're close enough to the forest to provide a sense of solitude, but their position facing the field gives campers a dramatic view of the hilltop, wildflowers, and trees, plus a sweeping expanse of sky. Most of these sites also give you a vista of the field on the hilltop from the front of the site and South Pond from the back. The pond isn't too close, but you can catch glimpses of it through the trees. The trail to South Pond Beach starts right between sites 17 and 18.

The spacious site 21 is tucked into a clearing in the dense forest at the end of this part of the campground loop road. Its position at the end of the road and the thick forest encircling the site give you a nice sense of solitude. The forest is also clear directly overhead, providing you with a good view of the night sky.

On the corner where the campground road loops around, site 22 is a bit more open but also roomy. Site 23, next door, is large and scenic. A grand old maple hovers overhead, offering a comfortable roof of sorts.

Nestled into a grove of small apple trees and wildflowers off the outer perimeter of the campground loop road, site 29 also has an orchard quality. It's also across from a water spigot. The other sites along this stretch of road are spacious and accessible but set apart and tucked into the woods enough to offer a bit of privacy.

The day-use area, down the road from the campground, has a beach and boat launch, giving you access to North Pond. Because of the easier access, expect North Pond to be more crowded than its sibling to the south. South Pond has a small beach area, but you can get there only through the campground. Both ponds have excellent hiking trails that loop around them and head toward the rest of Savoy Mountain State Forest's trail network.

MAP

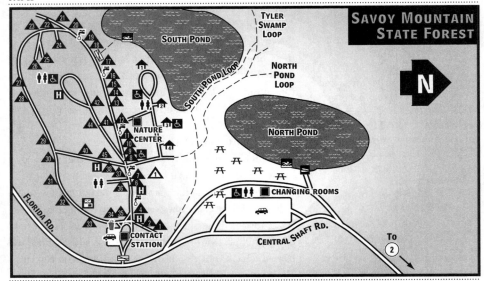

GETTING THERE

Follow MA 2 East into the town of Florida. Turn right on Central Shaft Road and follow the signs to Savoy Mountain State Forest.

GPS COORDINATES

N42° 38.921120'
W73° 2.815819'

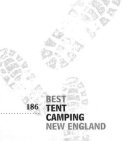

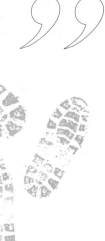

> *"Shawme-Crowell State Forest is another spot on Cape Cod where you can find a corner of the forest all for yourself."*

TUCKED INTO A CORNER of the beautiful town of Sandwich, Shawme-Crowell State Forest is the oldest campground and state forest in Massachusetts. You might just miss it altogether if you weren't looking for it specifically. The relative subtlety of its location is one reason that this is another of those spots on otherwise-crowded Cape Cod where you can always find a measure of solitude.

The other reason is its size. The campground has two main areas, each fairly large in its own right. There are 285 sites here at Shawme-Crowell State Forest. Overall, the size and composition of the sites is fairly uniform. There's also a good, hard sandy surface throughout all the sites for securing your tent stakes—no special wooden tent platforms needed here.

There is also a fairly uniform quality to the nature of the forest, although in certain areas the undergrowth is thicker and other areas are covered by towering groves of white pine. The mostly dense forest provides a decent overall sense of seclusion and shade to both camping areas 1 and 2.

In camping area 1, sites B2 through B5 are set up on a short spur off the B campground road. This is a great group of sites. You'll find quite a few site groupings like this at Shawme-Crowell State Forest: short roads leading off the main campground road, with two to four sites arranged in a small cluster. The sites on these short spurs are often somewhat open to each other but spectacularly secluded from their neighbors.

Site B1 and B6 are huge. The forest is very dense here at the ground level, so there's a fair degree of seclusion and a fairly consistent character to the sites throughout the B road.

As you move onto the C road, sites C2 through C4 make up another group of sites set off on their own road. Sites C6 through C8 are similarly grouped on their own

RATINGS

Beauty: ☆☆☆☆☆
Privacy: ☆☆☆
Spaciousness: ☆☆☆☆
Quiet: ☆☆☆☆
Security: ☆☆☆☆
Cleanliness: ☆☆☆☆☆

road. These small groups of sites offer a superb sense of seclusion. Another spectacularly secluded site is site C14, situated way off on its own.

The most exceptional sites here at Shawme-Crowell State Forest are those on the outer perimeter, on the outside of the primary campground loop roads, particularly those on the multiple short roads that lead off the main loop. There's a lush, almost primeval feeling to the forest here with lots of vines and other undergrowth, all tangled amid the classic low, scraggly Cape Cod forest.

Next on the C road are a couple more exceptional pairs of sites. Sites C18 and C19 are set up on a ridge, off on their own for a great sense of seclusion. Site C19 has a nice open view to the sky, while C18 is a bit more shaded. The pair of C21 and C22 is similar, with C21 being the more shaded of the two.

Sites C25 and C26 are also set off on their own. They're a bit more open to each other than some of the other pairs, so this would make a good pair of sites for a larger family or group. This pair, as well as sites 30 and 31, sit on a small ridge, so you'll frequently feel a breeze blowing through.

Next on the C road is a short loop with sites C32 through C36. While site C36 is fairly well secluded, the rest of the sites are open to each other. If you're camping with several families, these sites would be ideal. The rest of the sites toward the end of the C road—numbered on the high 40s—are a bit more open to each other and to the campground road.

Over on the E road, cutting through the center of camping area 1, sites E1 through E5 are a nice group, especially sites E3, E4, and E5. These sites are spaced farther up on a small hill, which gives them a solid sense of seclusion. Site E6 is also situated well off on its own.

Sites E9 through E11 form another nice group. Within this group, sites E10 and E11 are the best. Site E13 is close to the bathrooms, which may be good for some, but I prefer a bit more distance.

The D road also intersects camping area 1. There's a perfect sense of seclusion to sites D10 and D11, as these two are set up off of the road on their own. Site D8 is open and not very private, but it is quite spacious and scenic. This site also backs up against sites B9 through B11, so

MAP

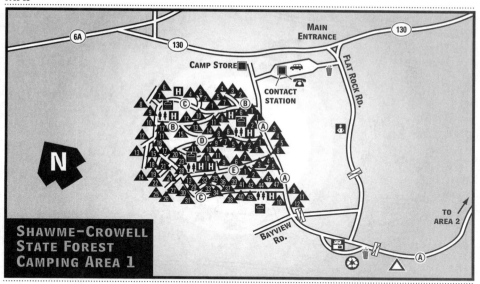

SHAWME-CROWELL
STATE FOREST
CAMPING AREA 1

GETTING THERE

Take US 6 East onto
Cape Cod to Exit 2 for
MA 130. Follow MA 130
through the center of Sandwich, then look for the sign
for Shawme-Crowell State
Forest on the left, 3 miles
past the center of Sandwich.

GPS COORDINATES

N41° 45.760682'
W70° 31.076703'

all of these sites feel very open. Sites B13 through B15 form another group of sites set on their own short road. These sites lie well back within a dense forest, especially site B14.

Heading out of camping area 1 and over to area 2 on the A road, you'll pass a beautiful, stately forest of tall white pine trees on your left. Farther down the A road into area 2, you'll see the first group site on your right. Shortly thereafter, the A road forks to the right. There on the left, you'll pass several of Shawme-Crowell State Forest's yurt sites.

As you move along the A road, sites A22 through A26 are a nice group of sites off on their own. Site A32 is also well secluded, set right where the fire road leads off of the campground A road.

The A road intersects the C road. The lower-numbered C-road sites are nicely spaced apart from each other, but the forest feels a bit more open at the forest-floor level. Site C3 is nice, set up off the road on a small ledge on the right. It's fairly open to sites C2 and C3, but this is a very scenic area of the forest.

As in camping area 1, the best sites in camping area 2 are those on the short roads leading off the main road.

MAP

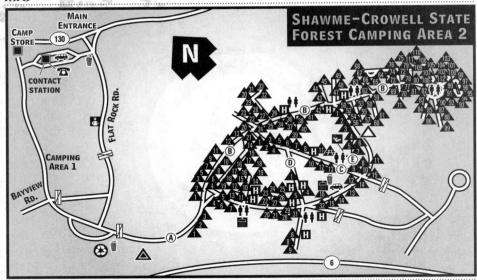

Many such groups of sites lie off the main B road leading deeper into area 2. Sites B26 through B33 feel a bit more open to each other at ground level, but they're covered by a tall, beautiful forest canopy of white pine. The forest is certainly older growth on this side of the campground.

Sites B52 through B57 are set within a dense, dark, cool grove of spruce and other conifers. Sites B62 and B63 are also nicely secluded from the road, if not from each other.

The group of sites including B64 through B68 is set well off on its own, right at the state-forest border. These sites are fairly open to each other, but the area feels like its own little campground. The grouping of sites B72 through B76 has a similar feel. Near site 77, a trailhead leads off to the rest of the network of hiking trails that wind through Shawme-Crowell State Forest.

As you move past these groups, the forest grows more dense—at least at the level of the forest floor. This imparts a nice sense of seclusion from neighboring sites—especially the sites on the short spur roads that lead off the loop at the end of the B road, like spokes on a bicycle. The site arrangement, combined with the more dense forest undergrowth, gives all these sites a decent sense of seclusion. These "spokes" include the B sites in the upper 80s, 90s, and 100s.

It's a large campground on the Cape, but you can still find plenty of spots within Shawme-Crowell State Forest that afford a sense of solitude—and that's why we set off with our tents in the first place.

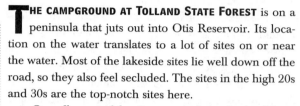

51
TOLLAND
STATE FOREST

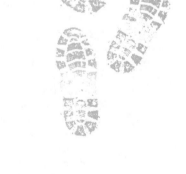

"Tolland State Forest has a bounty of waterfront sites—that magic combination of woods and water."

THE CAMPGROUND AT **TOLLAND STATE FOREST** is on a peninsula that juts out into Otis Reservoir. Its location on the water translates to a lot of sites on or near the water. Most of the lakeside sites lie well down off the road, so they also feel secluded. The sites in the high 20s and 30s are the top-notch sites here.

Overall, most of the sites are moderate in size. There are also a few management sites, designated by letters, spread throughout the campground (see map, page 193). These sites rotate in and out of circulation to minimize impact on the campground overall.

As you enter the outer campground loop, you'll find the lower-numbered sites starting on the right, facing the reservoir. You'll also find a couple of higher-numbered sites from where the road loops back, so sites 1 and 45 are across the road from each other. Site 46 is also near the entry to the campground. It's small and very open to the road, but because it's surrounded by beautiful dense forest, it feels more secluded at night.

Many of the lakeside sites are arranged in groups of three on short driveways that extend down toward the water from the main road. They're set mostly in a loosely spaced forest of pine and hemlock. Sites 2 and 3 are set a bit farther back from the road than site 1. Site 2 is fairly secluded, and site 3 is a bit more so. They're open to each other, though. A dense forest isolates these two sites from the road.

Sites 4, 5, and 6 encompass another cluster of sites that are open to each other but nicely secluded from any others. Because they're set in a fairly dense pine grove, they don't feel as open to the lake, although the lake is right there for easy access. Site 7 is well secluded on the sides but feels a bit open to the road.

The next cluster of sites includes sites 8, 9, and 10. Site 8 is closer to the road and a bit more open to it, but you'll enjoy good views of the lake through the trees. Sites

RATINGS

Beauty: ☆☆☆☆☆
Privacy: ☆☆☆☆
Spaciousness: ☆☆☆
Quiet: ☆☆☆
Security: ☆☆☆
Cleanliness: ☆☆☆☆

9 and 10 are down a bit farther, with great views of the lake from both sites, although they're open to each other. They'd be great for a larger group or family.

Another of Tolland State Forest's top-notch sites is site 12. A long driveway leads down to it, and it's right on the water. Sites 13, 14, and 15 are up off the lake. Site 16 is the site you'd want in this cluster.

The next trio of sites on the lake side of the campground road includes sites 18, 19, and 20. Of these three, site 18 is up a bit farther off the lake. Sites 19 and 20 are much closer, with commanding views and lake access.

Site 22, up a bit higher from the lake and closer to the road, has a bit more of an open feel, with sunlight filtering down through the trees. It's also across from the bathroom building. Site 21 is set in a beautiful pine grove but is also open to the road and to the restroom.

A long driveway leads into site 23 and a fairly dense forest on either side, so this stellar site has a nicely secluded feel. The fact that it's right on the lake puts it over the top for me. Site 24 has a shorter driveway leading into it and sits on a small rise overlooking the lake.

There's a bit more of an open feel to site 25, but you're on the lake. Sites 27 and 28 share a driveway. Site 27 is nicely secluded in a slightly denser forest. It's a bit farther down from the road and closer to the lake. Sites 29 and 30 are off on their own. Although they're open to the road and the restroom, they're set down off the road and near the lake. That's a tradeoff I'd be willing to make.

There's a small cul-de-sac at the end of the campground road here, with the sites spread out like spokes on a bike. Site 31 is down off the road close to the lake. Sites 32, 37, and 38 are open to the road and to each other, but again, they're right near the water. Sites 33, 34, and 35 are well off the road down close to the lakeshore. This is definitely where you want to be at this end of the campground.

There's a huge rock and stump in the center of site 39—a bit of natural landscaping. It's open to the sky and a bit open to the road, but very scenic. Sites 42 and 43 share a driveway, but site 43 feels more isolated. You have a short walk into 43, which is surrounded on all sides by forest. Site 42 is a bit smaller and more open.

KEY INFORMATION

ADDRESS:	410 Tolland Rd. P.O. Box 342 East Otis, MA 01029
OPERATED BY:	Massachusetts Department of Conservation and Recreation
INFORMATION:	413-269-6002
OPEN:	Late May– early Oct.
SITES:	94
EACH SITE:	Fire ring, picnic table
ASSIGNMENT:	First-come, first-served or by reservation: 877-422-6762, reserve america.com
REGISTRATION:	At ranger station as you enter campground
FACILITIES:	Flush toilets, showers, boat launch
PARKING:	At campsites
FEE:	Massachusetts residents, $12; non-residents, $14
RESTRICTIONS:	*Pets:* Dogs on leash only *Fires:* In established fire rings *Alcohol:* Prohibited *Vehicles:* Park at campsites *Other:* Reservations require 2-night minimum stay; campground office hours 8:30 a.m.–10 p.m.; 14-day maximum stay

MAP

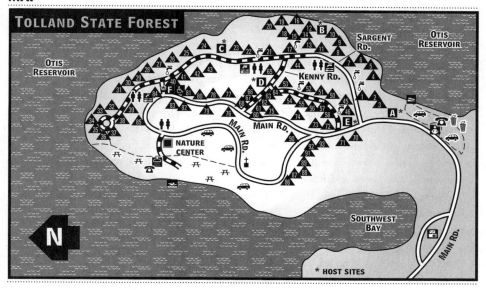

TOLLAND STATE FOREST

OTIS RESERVOIR

SARGENT RD.

OTIS RESERVOIR

KENNY RD.

MAIN RD.

NATURE CENTER

SOUTHWEST BAY

MAIN RD.

N

* HOST SITES

GETTING THERE

From the Massachusetts Turnpike (US 90), take Exit 3 in Westfield. Follow US 10/202 South 3 miles into downtown Westfield. Turn right onto US 20 West and continue 6 miles. Turn left onto MA 23 West and continue 11 miles through Blandford into Otis. About 0.5 mile past East Otis village, turn left at West Shore Road and follow the signs (West Shore Road becomes Reservoir Road). Turn left at Tolland Road and continue 2.2 miles to the campground.

The higher-numbered sites, in the 50s, 60s, and 70s, are in the interior of the peninsula, along Dean Road, Kenny Road, and the Main Road, respectively. Sites 50 and 51 have a bit more privacy than 52 through 55, but they're still fairly open to the road and to each other. Sites 52, 53, 54, and 55 are very open to the road and to each other. They're beautiful sites, though, and they're in a quiet corner of the campground.

Sunlight filters down to the forest floor in site 56, which is open to the sky and encircled by towering pines. Sites 57 and 58 are set down off the road and so might grant you a bit more seclusion.

Site 60 is a bit smaller but fairly well secluded. It's surrounded by towering hardwoods and dense undergrowth at the back. Sites 61, 62, 66, and 67 are smaller. They're moderately well secluded on the sides but quite open to the road and to each other. Site 63 is set apart for greater privacy.

GPS COORDINATES

N42° 8.651576'
W73° 2.656095'

If you need a huge site, check out site 64. The tradeoff is that it's very open to the road. Site 65 is a good-sized site that's well off on its own, but it's completely open to the bathroom at the back of the site. That's too bad, because it's awesome otherwise. Site 68 is very spacious. It's open to the road and the sky above, but there's a dense forest to the back and sides.

Sites 70 and 71 are well away from other sites but fairly open to each other. A huge white pine stands the center of site 72. It's a smaller site, though, and very open to the road. Site 73 is also fairly open to the road and sits at an intersection, but it's secluded alongside and behind.

You'll get a spectacular sense of isolation at sites 74 and 75, even though they're close to each other. Site 74 is set back off the road and carved out of the dense forest. It's very picturesque, with shards of sunlight filtering down. Site 75 is smaller and closer to the road, yet well isolated and scenic. You could almost picture sitting there with the members of the Fellowship discussing how to get into Mordor.

While sites 77 and 76 are off on their own, they're also very open to the road at an intersection of the campground roads. Site 79 is huge site in a majestic stand of towering birch and pine, so it's nicely shaded. It has an open feel, but it's very picturesque.

Right on the lake at Southwest Bay, sites 87 and 86 are secluded and offer water views and access. Sites 82 and 83 are very open to the road and to each other. These would make a good pair of sites for a larger group. Likewise with sites 80, 81, and 78. The forest is more loosely spaced here, with a bit less undergrowth. This contributes to an open and airy feel but affords much less privacy.

Sites 89 and 88 offer only moderate seclusion. They're a bit open to the road and to each other. Site 90 is a bit more secluded, surrounded by a younger forest of smaller trees. Site 91 is a bright, sunny site framed by massive white pines.

There's a funky white pine with multiple trunks just beside site 93, which gives it a unique character. The kid in me can't help but imagine what a wild tree house you could build here.

The forest here is fairly dense for the most part, adding to the sense of seclusion, even for sites that are a bit more open to each other, like sites 52 through 55. There is some boat noise during the day, but it's quiet at night. The juxtaposition of woods and water is always a powerful combination. Do what you can to get a waterfront site when you come to Tolland State Forest. The effort is worth it.

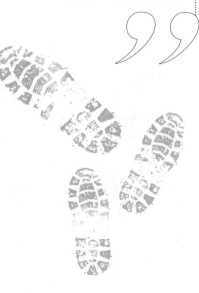

> *Washburn Island feels as wild and remote as somewhere in the South Pacific—but getting there is much easier.*

REMOTE, UNCROWDED, QUIET—words not often associated with Cape Cod, especially during the crazy summer season. Washburn Island may change the way you look at the Cape. It certainly did for me. The island is right at the mouth of the Childs River. When you paddle or motor out there, you're never too far from shore. Plus, these are protected waters that rarely get too rough, so it would be a relatively easy trip if you plan to arrive by canoe or kayak, making this is a perfect spot for your first island camping experience.

Long, sweeping, flat, and sandy, the beach opens to a shallow bay with gentle waves. This would be a very safe place for kids to spend the day in and out of the water, which tends to be a bit warmer here as it's so shallow.

The campsites on Washburn Island are all spectacularly secluded. There truly isn't a bad site here. This is a pack-in, pack-out camping area, meaning you have to take out all your trash. Also, there are no open fires or fire rings. You'll have to do your cooking on a portable hibachi or campstove. You'll also have to bring all your own water, as there are no water sources on the island.

Hike up toward the manager's tent behind the informational signs posted on the beach as you arrive, then turn right on the trail to get to sites 1 through 6, or left to get to sites 7 through 10. Site 9 is the group site. All are marked (from both the inland side and from the beach) by small painted stones.

Sites 1 and 2 would be perfect for a group wanting two contiguous spots. Site 1 is a bit smaller than 2, but similar in character in that a dense wall of forest runs behind and alongside, with an open view of the beach to the front.

Up on a small bluff overlooking the beach, site 2 has a truly dazzling view of the bay. There's also a nice sense of seclusion to this site, as it has dense forest and undergrowth running alongside. Site 2 is fairly close to site 1,

RATINGS

Beauty: ✰ ✰ ✰ ✰ ✰
Privacy: ✰ ✰ ✰ ✰ ✰
Spaciousness: ✰ ✰ ✰ ✰ ✰
Quiet: ✰ ✰ ✰ ✰ ✰
Security: ✰ ✰ ✰ ✰ ✰
Cleanliness: ✰ ✰ ✰ ✰ ✰

but both are separated from the rest of the campsites, if not from each other.

Site 3 is a good size. It's relatively close to the bathroom building on the eastern side of the campground, but not too close. As it's a larger site, this would be a good one for a large family or group. Sites 4, 5, and 6 are all fairly open to each other but still quite spectacular. Sites 5 and 6 are moderately spacious, with lots of trees sprinkled throughout. They are both very open to the beach.

Spread out along the southwestern shore of the island, sites 7 through 10 all open to the beach. Sites 7 and 8 are a bit closer to each other, but that certainly doesn't detract from their magnificence. They're still secluded by the forest, and also perched a bit higher off the beach. Sites 7 and 8 are moderate in size, similar to site 10, which is more isolated.

If stargazing is your thing, check out group site 9. It's very open to the sky and it funnels right down to the beach. You'll have plenty of room to set up your tent anywhere you want within this site. Its size makes it suitable for a larger group or family.

Site 10 feels incredibly remote, surrounded by 50-foot-tall scrubby white pines and maples. The ground on this site, and most of the others, is a firm, sandy surface covered by a blanket of pine needles. The loosely spaced forest opens to the bay for a million-dollar view of the water and cool sea breezes—a truly magical combination.

The paths within the sites and the hiking trails leading around the island are all very well marked with neatly arranged fallen limbs. Please stay on the paths when walking about the island to preserve its fragile ecology. You'll also reduce the danger of picking up a tick, which is a real possibility here. Check yourself and your kids thoroughly. If you find one, don't panic. Ticks have to be embedded for about 24 hours to transmit disease. If you check yourself every day, you should be fine.

The openness to the beach, the incredible views, and the sense of seclusion in most of the campsites are a powerful combination. The silence is remarkable, especially for the Cape. Were the pines and beech trees on Washburn Island suddenly replaced by palm trees, you'd swear you were somewhere in the South Pacific.

KEY INFORMATION

ADDRESS:	P.O. Box 3092 149 Waquoit Hwy. Waquoit, MA 02536
OPERATED BY:	Massachusetts Department of Conservation and Recreation
INFORMATION:	508-457-0495, waquoitbay reserve.org
OPEN:	Early May– early Oct.
SITES:	9 plus 1 group site
EACH SITE:	Incredible beauty
ASSIGNMENT:	By reservation only: 877-422-6762, reserve america.com)
REGISTRATION:	Camping permit required
FACILITIES:	Composting toilets; no water available, so bring plenty
PARKING:	On the beach!
FEE:	Massachusetts residents, $6; nonresidents, $8; group site, $25
RESTRICTIONS:	*Pets:* Dogs on leash at sites, prohibited on beach *Fires:* No open fires; use portable grills or stoves only *Alcohol:* Not allowed *Vehicles:* Pull your canoe or kayak up on the beach *Other:* 5 people maximum per campsite, 25 maximum for group site, pack out all trash, check in after 1 p.m., check out by 11 a.m.

MAP

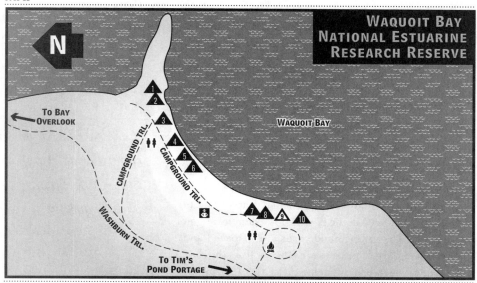

GETTING THERE

From Falmouth, head south on MA 28 and park at the White's Landing boat launch, next to Bosun's Marine (formerly Edwards Boatyard). Paddle out of the Childs River, bear left, and follow the shoreline of Washburn Island to the campsites.

GPS COORDINATES

N41° 33.814359'
W70° 31.788640'

THERE ARE TWO SIDES to the campground at Wompatuck State Park: electric and nonelectric. Obviously, the nonelectric side is going to be the one with the best tent camping. The forest here is fairly dense with birch, maple, sumac, and pine. Generally, it's nice and quiet—all you'll hear is the breeze rustling through the trees.

The sites are numbered and lettered according to the road they're on. All the N sites, for example, are on the N road. The campground roads are all paved and well marked. Most of the sites are set back from the road at an angle, which helps increase the sense of seclusion.

The nonelectric side has the N-through-Y sites. The layout and letter–number designation can be a bit confusing, so have a campground map handy as you read this profile when you're making your plans. (Go to **tinyurl.com/wompcamp**.)

Despite being near an intersection of the campground road, site N2 is well secluded. Although slightly smaller, it has a short berm at the end that affords some privacy. N3 is also well secluded. Sites N4 and N5 are blocked on the sides yet fairly open to each other.

N19, another small site, is also well secluded on the sides, even though it's open to an intersection of the campground roads. Similarly, N17 and N18 are very secluded on the sides, although a bit open to each other.

The forest opens a bit more around N17. This site also has an old stone wall running along its border. N15 is very large and feels a bit more open as the forest is quite loosely spaced behind. N13 is nicely secluded on the sides, yet somewhat open to the loosely spaced forest toward the back.

Sites N11 and N10 are both fairly private. N11 is a smaller site, but nicely secluded on all sides. Site N10 is surrounded by mixed forest. Site N9 is a slightly smaller site, but the dense mixed forest protects the back and sides.

> *The dense forest gives the campsites at Wompatuck State Park a cool, woodsy quality.*

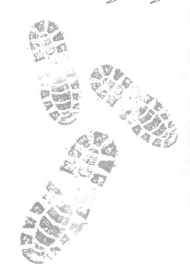

RATINGS

Beauty: ✩ ✩ ✩ ✩
Privacy: ✩ ✩ ✩ ✩
Spaciousness: ✩ ✩ ✩ ✩
Quiet: ✩ ✩ ✩ ✩
Security: ✩ ✩ ✩ ✩
Cleanliness: ✩ ✩ ✩ ✩

KEY INFORMATION

ADDRESS: Union Street Hingham, MA 02043

OPERATED BY: Massachusetts Department of Conservation and Recreation

INFORMATION: 781-749-7160 (in season), 781-749-7161 (year-round)

OPEN: Early May– mid-Oct.

SITES: 261 (150 on non-electric side, 111 on electric side)

EACH SITE: Fire ring, picnic table

ASSIGNMENT: First-come, first-served or by reservation: 877-422-6762, reserve america.com

REGISTRATION: At ranger station as you enter campground

FACILITIES: Flush toilets, hot showers

PARKING: At campsites

FEE: Massachusetts residents, $12; nonresidents, $14

RESTRICTIONS: *Pets:* Dogs on leash only
Fires: In established fire rings
Alcohol: Prohibited
Vehicles: Park at campsites
Other: Reservations require 2-night minimum stay; campground-office hours 8 a.m.– 10 p.m.; 14-day maximum stay

Now on to the sites on the O road. Site O1 has a nice grassy surface and is smaller but well secluded. Site O3 is separated by the dense forest. Farther along the O road, the woods get a bit more open, so generally there's less privacy. Sites O4 and O5, for example, have a loosely spaced forest alongside. Site O8 has even less seclusion because the forest is so sparse, but it's very scenic nonetheless.

Site O12 is large. It's also open to the sky, so it's quite sunny during the day. There's a nice sense of seclusion to site O15, as the forest fills in here. It's also set off on the outside of a bend in the campground road. Site O15 is also quite large and private.

The *P* in the P road must stand for *primeval,* as the area is dense with forest, ferns, and thick pines. Sites P1 and P3 are a good size, but they're a bit open to the road and to each other. P4 is a much smaller site that also has a fairly open feel. P6 is a nice big site. The forest is fairly loose here, but it's still a secluded site. A little berm blocks the site from the road.

Set in a loosely spaced grove of pines, P8 is a good-sized site. It has a bit of an open feel, though, so you'd probably see your neighbors on the Q road through the forest. P14 is small but very well secluded on the sides. Sites P16 and P9 are smaller sites as well, but a grove of young maple provides privacy. Site P18 is moderate in size and very well secluded, even though it's near a campground road intersection.

Most of the Q sites have an open feel. Q1 and Q2 are both very open to the road and bathroom building at the intersection of the campground roads, so those afford a bit less privacy, although they are convenient to the restroom.

Q3 is long and narrow, so it gets fairly secluded deeper into the site. Site Q4 is much smaller and is framed by towering pines, so it's scenic albeit a bit open to the road. Site Q6 is a huge site and fairly secluded alongside and behind, but again it's a bit open to the road. On the other hand, Q5 is much smaller yet more private.

Site Q8 is more secluded still because there's more space between the neighboring sites on that side of the campground road. Site Q7, Q9, and Q10 feel private but are all in very loosely spaced forest.

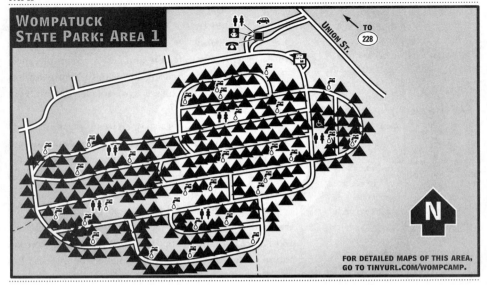

WOMPATUCK STATE PARK: AREA 1

TO 228

UNION ST.

N

FOR DETAILED MAPS OF THIS AREA, GO TO TINYURL.COM/WOMPCAMP.

Even though it's at an intersection, Q17 is fairly secluded on the sides. Site Q19 is huge. It's set in a loose forest but is still isolated. Sites Q20 and Q21 are a bit smaller and protected on the sides but open to the road. Good-sized and very secluded, site Q22 sits at a bend in the road. Beyond that is a closed area of the campground.

Along the R road, you'll find a prime site right off the bat. R2 is beautiful and quite spacious, set in a grove of young white pines, with a small berm defining the back of the site.

R3 is small but private. Both R4 and R5 have a much more open feel; R4 is the much larger of the two. Sites R6 and R7 are both secluded on the sides and back yet open to each other across the road. They make for a nice pair if you're camping with a larger group. Likewise with R8 and R9—private yet open to each other across the road. R11 is a smaller site with lots of privacy. It's also much more open to the sky than the other R sites. Site R13 is medium-sized with a nice sense of seclusion, as there's no site across the road.

GETTING THERE

From MA 3, take Exit 14. Then follow MA 228 North about 5 miles to Free Street. Turn right on Free Street and go 1 mile to the park entrance on Union Street, on the right. Follow Union Street 1.5 miles to the campground entrance, also on the right.

GPS COORDINATES

N42° 12.178838'
W70° 50.806353'

Sites R10 through R15 all have a very open feel. They abut a closed area, though, so you won't have as many neighbors. Sites R12 and R17 also have a very open feel as they're set in a young, loosely spaced forest. This is a quiet corner of the campground.

A few T-lettered sites lie at the end of the R road. T1 and T2 are very nicely secluded, off near the end of the open area of the campground.

The X road is home to a few smaller but private sites. Site X15 is very shaded and secluded on the sides. X13 is a bit smaller, set near what's left of an old stone wall that gives it some character. This site is also very private. X8 and X11 are fairly open to the road but separated from each other.

Site X6 is a bit smaller, very shaded, and fairly open to the road. It also has the old stone wall defining its edge. Sites X7 and X5 are also small, secluded, and shaded—framed by the towering forest and filled in with dense undergrowth.

On the Y road, Y1 is set within a towering pine grove but right across from the restroom. Y4 is much more open to the road and to the bathroom, although it's a good size.

Site Y5 is moderately sized, framed by pines and maples. It's a bit open to the road but secluded on the sides. Site Y9, very spacious and open, is framed by the forest, with sunlight filtering through. Y7 is fairly secluded on the sides. Though it feels a bit open at the back, it's mostly open to the forest.

When you come to Wompatuck State Park, be sure to bring your bike—especially if you're a mountain biker. Miles of trails wind through the park, awaiting your exploration.

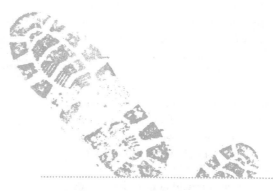

CONNECTICUT

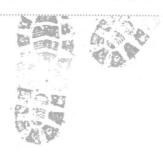

54
DEVIL'S HOPYARD STATE PARK

IF YOU'RE WONDERING HOW THIS state park came by its name, you're not alone. A variety of theories exist. One thing folks do agree on is that the name refers to the numerous holes bored into the rock at the base of Chapman Falls. The most oft-repeated "explanation" is that these are the result of the devil hopping from rock to rock to avoid getting his hooves wet, burning holes in the rocks with each hop. If you can think of a better or more entertaining theory, feel free to share it with your fellow campers.

The Chapman Falls Campground at Devil's Hopyard State Park has 22 sites spread out in a wooded grove right near the campground's namesake. The falls not only provide a beautiful spot to relax and enjoy the view right outside the campground, but the constant rush of the water is a welcome addition to the forest's soundtrack.

The wooded sites at this cozy little campground are arranged on either side of the short campground road. The sites are spacious but not too private. A barrier of scrub brush separates the campground from the waters above Chapman Falls on one side; on the other side, the sites abut the woods.

The sites along the water are pleasant. Those at the end of the loop are even nicer, and they have the added benefit of being a bit more private. Site 8 is one of the more secluded sites in the campground. Sites 10 and 11 are also set off from the rest of the campground but not from each other. This would be a good pair of sites for a group.

Site 15 is desirable, as it's right along the water leading to the falls. Sites 16, 17, and 18 are all incredibly peaceful places to camp right along the water. Site 16 is the key spot for anglers—you could fish right from your campsite (for information on fishing licenses, see Appendix C, page 232).

> *Devil's Hopyard is small and scenic, with a cozy group of campsites just a few steps from Chapman Falls.*

RATINGS

Beauty: ☆ ☆ ☆ ☆ ☆
Privacy: ☆ ☆ ☆
Spaciousness: ☆ ☆ ☆ ☆
Quiet: ☆ ☆ ☆ ☆ ☆
Security: ☆ ☆ ☆ ☆ ☆
Cleanliness: ☆ ☆ ☆ ☆

Because of its small size and remote location, the campground is very quiet except for the welcome sounds of the woodland birds and the light, incessant rushing of Chapman Falls. The loosely spaced forest of mixed deciduous and coniferous trees lets in a lot of light. The forest at the border of the campground and within the rest of the park is much more densely packed.

Chapman Falls is a spectacular series of waterfalls cascading nearly 60 feet and continuing on as the Eight-mile River. The river flows past the Devil's Hopyard picnic area a bit farther downstream from the campground. This day-use area is popular with anglers; it's also a scenic place to walk around or just relax. Except for the campground, Devil's Hopyard State Park is closed from sunset to 6 a.m.

This area of Connecticut is just north of the town of Lyme. If that name sounds familiar, it should: Lyme has the unique and unwelcome distinction of being home to the first diagnosed cases of Lyme disease. While incidences of the disease are now documented all across the United States, it's still worth keeping an especially keen eye out for deer ticks in this area. Nymph (baby) deer ticks are particularly nasty and are extremely small and difficult to find. This doesn't mean you should stay inside all summer long—just check yourself very carefully, especially your head and hair. If you do find a tick, don't panic. Generally, the tick has to be embedded for 24 hours to transmit the disease. Remove the tick completely with a pair of tweezers, and sterilize the bite with an antiseptic first-aid ointment.

MAP

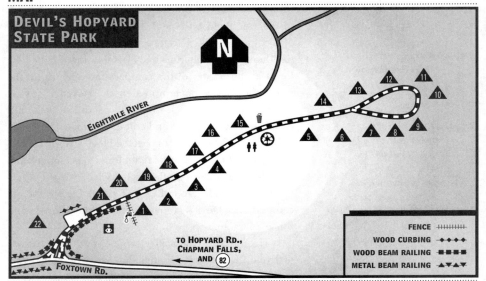

DEVIL'S HOPYARD
STATE PARK

N

EIGHTMILE RIVER

FENCE	+++++++
WOOD CURBING	◆◆◆◆
WOOD BEAM RAILING	■■■■
METAL BEAM RAILING	▲▼▲▼

TO HOPYARD RD.,
CHAPMAN FALLS,
AND (82)

FOXTOWN RD.

GETTING THERE

From the intersection of
CT 82 and CT 154, follow
Hopyard Road north about
3 miles. Turn right on
Foxtown Road and follow
it to the campground,
on your left.

GPS COORDINATES

N41° 29.049489'
W72° 20.506182'

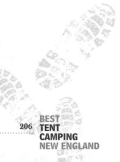

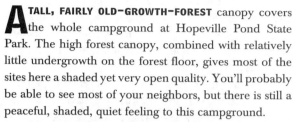

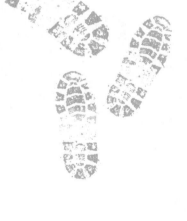

The placid waters of Hopeville Pond make this a worthwhile destination for a few days of camping and fishing.

A TALL, FAIRLY OLD-GROWTH-FOREST canopy covers the whole campground at Hopeville Pond State Park. The high forest canopy, combined with relatively little undergrowth on the forest floor, gives most of the sites here a shaded yet very open quality. You'll probably be able to see most of your neighbors, but there is still a peaceful, shaded, quiet feeling to this campground.

Most of the A and B sites are fairly open and fairly uniform in size. The higher-numbered B sites are very open yet have a bit more sunlight filtering down to the sites. Shady, open sites abound in the A and B areas of the campground. Sites B1 through B3 are very open and close to the bathrooms.

At the end of the B and C loops, the sites are near the shores of Hopeville Pond. This is where you want to be—close to the pond, with at the very least a decent view of the pond through the trees. In this part of the campground, sites B12 and B10 are nicely shaded yet still have a fairly open feeling to them.

It's very quiet here. The campground is far enough from any major roads that it gets hardly any road noise. There are no sites right on the pond per se, but they are very close. The pond is across the campground road from many of the B and C sites. It's definitely worth trying to find a site in this part of the campground.

Moving along the outside of the campground loop road brings you into the C area. Sites C9 and C11 are right next to the small beach and boat launch. The higher-numbered C sites are still very open at the ground level, yet they're nicely shaded above by the forest canopy and close to the shores of the pond.

At the end of the E road are some nice pondside sites—especially the E sites in the teens. The inner E and D loops are nicely shaded but very open at the ground level. For the best pond views and pond access, try to select a site on the outer side of the campground road.

RATINGS

Beauty: ✫ ✫ ✫ ✫
Privacy: ✫ ✫ ✫
Spaciousness: ✫ ✫ ✫ ✫
Quiet: ✫ ✫ ✫
Security: ✫ ✫ ✫ ✫
Cleanliness: ✫ ✫ ✫ ✫

While it's set back from the pond, site E1 is surprisingly spacious. It feels a bit more set off than the rest of the sites, as it's situated at the end of the campground road. This site is also right next to an open, grassy area that would be a good place for sunbathing, stargazing, or throwing around a football or Frisbee.

Overall, this campground is a bit more open than I typically prefer, but the statuesque forest canopy provides a nice cover of shade and quiet. And you can't beat being close to the pond. Woods and water are always a powerful combination.

On the other side of the campground, past the ranger building, is F Street, as the sign says. This is the small loop to the F sites—which were closed the last time I visited Hopeville Pond State Park. It was unclear whether they were closed for good or just closed early for the season. These are great, nicely secluded sites, though, so put in a call to the park to see if you can score one of them.

The forest in the F loop has a much more dense feeling than that in the rest of the campground. It also has much more undergrowth, which helps promote a greater sense of seclusion among the individual sites. Site F3 is fabulously isolated, yet a considerable amount of sunlight filters down to it.

At the back side of the loop, site F9 is nice but close to the bathroom. Sites F12 and F13 are set up on the outside of the loop. F12 is very open and sunny, while site F13 is a bit more shaded.

Hopeville Pond State Park is a nice, quiet, relaxing place. You should definitely try for one of the outer-rim sites so you're as close to the pond as possible.

KEY INFORMATION

ADDRESS: 193 Roode Rd. Jewett City, CT 06351

OPERATED BY: Connecticut Department of Energy and Environmental Protection

INFORMATION: 860-376-2920

OPEN: Mid-April–Sept. 30

SITES: 81

EACH SITE: Fire ring with grate, picnic table

ASSIGNMENT: First-come, first-served or by reservation: 860-376-0313

REGISTRATION: Hopeville Pond Campground

FACILITIES: Flush toilets, water spigots

PARKING: At sites

FEE: Connecticut residents, $17; non-residents, $27

RESTRICTIONS: *Pets:* Not allowed
Fires: Fire rings only
Alcohol: Prohibited
Vehicles: 1 per site
Other: Quiet hours 10 p.m.–7 a.m.

MAP

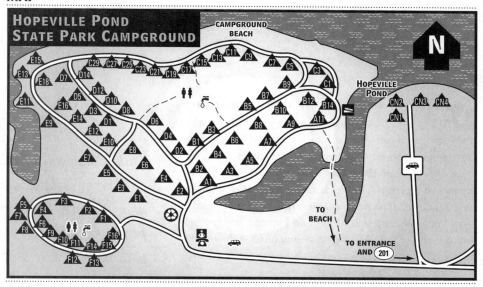

GETTING THERE

From I-395 (heading either north or south), take Exit 86. From the north, turn left off the exit; from the south, turn right. Follow Hopeville Road to the park signs. The park entrance is just off CT 201, on the right.

GPS COORDINATES

N41° 36.097677'
W71° 56.145236'

MACEDONIA BROOK STATE PARK

DEEP IN THE FORESTS OF WESTERN **CONNECTICUT,** Macedonia Brook State Park is grand in both size and character. Following the long access road leading into the campground—or more accurately, campgrounds, as there are several distinct areas within the park—you'll pass some stellar picnic areas set beneath the towering forest and right beside the pristine waters of Macedonia Brook. You'll also pass the sites of the Old Furnace, the Gorge, and the Lower Falls. Myriad twists and turns in the brook invite you to spend hours casting a line in the tumbling water to coax out a brook trout.

There are six separate camping areas within Macedonia Brook State Park: Birch, Hickory, Brookside, Red Pine, Overlook, and Maple. Some of these areas are further subdivided, and they're spread out along the long and winding road leading through the campground. The remote wilderness character of the forest, combined with the widely dispersed camping areas, gives the entire campground a quiet, secluded feeling.

You'll pass the day-use pavilion and volleyball net as you drive toward the camping areas, and the Silver Birch Area is the first group of campsites you'll come to. Sites 1 through 4 in Silver Birch are open sites within a grassy loop right by Macedonia Brook. While these sites don't offer much seclusion from one another, they are completely separate from the rest of the campground. Their riverside location is their most compelling characteristic. You could fly-fish right from your site (for information on fishing licenses, see Appendix C, page 232).

The Upper Birch Area includes sites 7 through 12, which are open, spacious, and neat but not particularly private. They sit on a grassy hillside with sporadic trees, but the whole area is surrounded by dense woods. Many of the sites border forest. The field offers sweeping views of the night sky for an intense stargazing experience. The constant whoosh of the stream rushing by is peaceful and

> *Macedonia Brook State Park is magically scenic, with many isolated sites along the river that are perfect for fishing or just watching the river flow.*

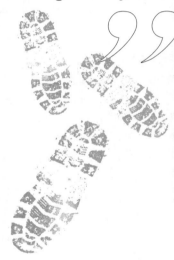

RATINGS

Beauty: ✰ ✰ ✰ ✰ ✰
Privacy: ✰ ✰ ✰ ✰
Spaciousness: ✰ ✰ ✰ ✰
Quiet: ✰ ✰ ✰ ✰ ✰
Security: ✰ ✰ ✰ ✰
Cleanliness: ✰ ✰ ✰ ✰ ✰

KEY INFORMATION

ADDRESS: 159 Macedonia Brook Rd. Kent, CT 06757

OPERATED BY: Connecticut Department of Energy and Environmental Protection

INFORMATION: 860-927-4100 (campground), 860-927-3238 (park office)

OPEN: Mid-April–Sept. 30

SITES: 51

EACH SITE: Fire ring or stone hearth, picnic table

ASSIGNMENT: First-come, first-served; by reservation mid-April–end of Sept.: 877-668-2267, reserveamerica.com

REGISTRATION: At ranger station

FACILITIES: Pit toilets

PARKING: At sites

FEE: Connecticut residents, $14; nonresidents, $24

RESTRICTIONS: *Pets:* Prohibited
Fires: In fire rings only
Alcohol: Prohibited
Vehicles: Parking at sites only
Other: Check out by noon; quiet hours 11 p.m.–7 a.m.; no swimming in river

relaxing. There is a water pump between sites 11 and 12, which also have huge stone hearths for your campfire instead of the typical fire ring.

The Lower Hickory Area includes sites 13 through 17. They're close to the river and fairly isolated, although the forest is open within this area. Upper Hickory is home to sites 21 and 22. These sites are even more exposed, set on the border between the forest and an open, grassy area.

The Red Pine Loop, with sites 24 through 27, is pleasantly isolated. I especially like this corner of the campground; there's not a bad spot here. The woods are a bit denser, so these sites offer a great sense of seclusion. There are more deciduous trees mixed into the forest, and the added shade gives these spots a deep-woods feel. Site 24 is tucked off on its own at the top of the loop, and site 25 is nicely isolated.

Perched on the banks of Macedonia Brook, the Brookside sites 28 and 29 would be well suited for a group wanting to fly-fish. These two sites sit together on a small grassy field right next to the brook. They're exposed—set between the brook and the campground road—but they actually become quite private later in the day, as they're entirely separated from the rest of the campground.

The Overlook Area includes sites 31 through 42. The upper sites on this wide, grassy hillside have a spectacular view of the forest, sky, and the surrounding hillsides of South Cobble and Chase mountains. The large sites within this loop aren't terribly private, though.

The Maple Area is quite spread out and includes sites 43 through 51. These sites are beautifully isolated in a dense grove of varied tree species. These loops are just past the Overlook Area as you drive along the campground road.

The camping areas within Macedonia Brook State Park seem to offer a choice between seclusion and sweeping views. The sites on the grassy hillsides are more open to breezes, so they're often cooler and less buggy than the sites set deep within the woods.

Numerous hiking trails wind throughout the state park, and campers have plenty of places to drop a hook in the water. Most of the trails are called (and marked)

MAP

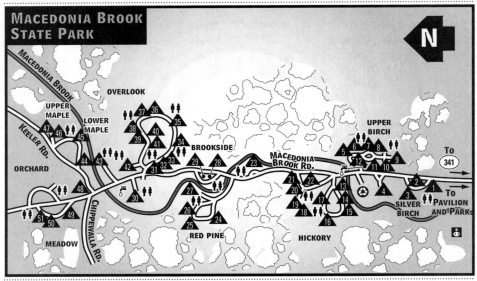

simply by colors. The Blue Trail follows a ridgeline to the east of the camping areas. The Yellow Trail intersects the Blue Trail just west of the pavilion. The Green Trail, leading out from the Upper Birch Area, also intersects the Blue Trail. The Orange Trail runs from the Upper Birch Area to the Maple Area. Lastly, the White Trail takes you from the pavilion to the top of nearby Cobble Mountain.

GETTING THERE

From Kent, follow CT 341 north to Macedonia Brook Road, on the right. Turn right here and drive until you see signs for the park.

GPS COORDINATES

N41° 45.972748'
W73° 29.695394'

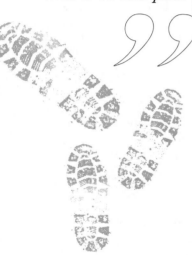

Of the two separate camping areas here, the one where you want to land is the Mashamoquet Brook Campground, closer to the state park.

PAY ATTENTION AS YOU APPROACH the Mashamoquet Brook State Park and campgrounds—there are three separate entrances for the state-park day-use area and hiking trails, the Mashamoquet Brook Campground, and the Wolf Den Campground. Each of these entrances is separated by a couple of miles along US 44. As you head west on US 44, you'll first come to the entrance for the Wolf Den Campground, which is actually marked as Wolf Den State Park. A couple miles farther down on the same side, you'll come to Mashamoquet Brook State Park. A couple more miles west brings you to the Mashamoquet Brook Campground—which is where you want to be when camping here.

This part of the campground is smaller and set within a beautiful dense forest. It gets a little bit of road noise from Route 44 during the day, as the campground is fairly close to the road, but that fades off at night.

Most of the sites here are moderately open to each other, as there is little undergrowth to the forest here. The sites on the right side of the campground road heading in are quite large.

As you enter the campground and bear off toward the left, sites 41 and 42 are the first sites you'll encounter. Site 41 is moderately sized, but site 42 is huge. Site 43 is another exceptionally large site. As you move farther down this side of the campground road, site 44 is another good-sized site.

Site 45 is huge as well. There's plenty of room here for a large tent or a couple of tents. This site is also set up off the campground road a bit. It's also right across from the bathroom, though—good for some, but I prefer to be a bit farther away. Two other sites that are quite large but feel very open are sites 46 and site 48.

On the other side of the road, site 57 is a bit smaller but more secluded on the sides. Site 60 is very open and sunny, surrounded by dense, mostly deciduous forest.

RATINGS

Beauty: ✰ ✰ ✰ ✰
Privacy: ✰ ✰ ✰
Spaciousness: ✰ ✰ ✰ ✰
Quiet: ✰ ✰ ✰
Security: ✰ ✰ ✰ ✰
Cleanliness: ✰ ✰ ✰ ✰

Site 59 is shaded by a towering hemlock tree. It's also close to the bathrooms.

The loop at the end of the campground road here has sites scattered along the outside of the loop, and a small, grassy field within. This would be a great spot for tossing a Frisbee or stargazing at night. Overall, these sites are clean and quiet and all fairly good-sized, although somewhat open to the road. The forest is a dense, lush mix of hardwoods and conifers, with sufficient sunlight filtering down to the forest floor.

There are no campsites within the Mashamoquet Brook State Park day-use area, but there are hiking trails leading from the campground to the day-use area. You'll also find spots for fishing and swimming. The forest and hiking trails here are exceptionally beautiful. You can hike from the Mashamoquet Brook Campground to the state park and day-use area.

Farther east on US 44, and on the same side of the road as the Mashamoquet Brook campground and state-park day-use area, is the Wolf Den camping area. Keep in mind that this is marked on US 44 as Wolf Den State Park, although all these areas operate under the auspices of Mashamoquet Brook State Park.

The turnoff for Wolf Den and the camping area is still a couple of miles farther down the road on the left. Overall, this camping area is much quieter than the Mashamoquet Brook Campground by virtue of its distance from Route 44. The entire campground, however, has a much more open, less private feeling.

Small, scattered clumps of trees provide some shade, and the sites are all quite uniform in size and orientation on both the inside and outside of the loop. These sites do feel very much like camping in an open field, though. Wolf Den is okay, but I much prefer the peacefulness of Mashamoquet Brook Campground. Whether you travel here for the hiking or fishing, you'll find a decent sense of solitude and some spectacularly beautiful forest here at Mashamoquet Brook State Park.

KEY INFORMATION

ADDRESS: US 44 Pomfret Center, CT 02659

OPERATED BY: Connecticut Department of Energy and Environmental Protection

INFORMATION: 860-928-6121

OPEN: Mid-April–Sept. 30

SITES: 18

EACH SITE: Fire ring with grate, picnic table

ASSIGNMENT: First-come, first-served or by reservation: 860-928-6121

REGISTRATION: Mashamoquet Brook State Park

FACILITIES: Flush and composting toilets, water spigots

PARKING: At sites

FEE: Connecticut residents, $14; non-residents, $24

RESTRICTIONS: *Pets:* Not allowed
Fires: Fire rings only
Alcohol: At sites only
Vehicles: 1 per site
Other: Quiet hours 10 p.m.–7 a.m.

MAP

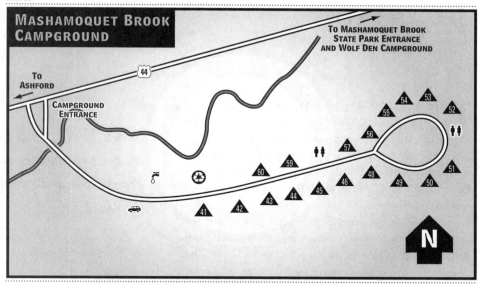

GETTING THERE

From I-395 (heading either north or south), take Exit 93. Turn onto CT 101 West. Follow CT 101 West until it joins US 44. Wolf Den Campground will be near the intersection of CT 101 and US 44. The state park and Mashamoquet Brook Campground will be another couple of miles to the west.

GPS COORDINATES

N41° 51.070561'
W71° 58.108921'

THERE IS ABSOLUTELY NO WAY you'll find an RV at the Selden Neck Campground, in Gillette Castle State Park. It has no designated tent-only areas, and no inherent rules or regulations prohibiting them, but until someone invents an RV that floats, Selden Neck is just for tent camping. You can reach the park and the campground only by boat.

This fabulously peaceful little state park is perched on the northern corner of a small island separated from the banks of the Connecticut River by Selden Creek. The campsites are right on the river, and there are no docks, moorings, or facilities other than fireplaces and pit toilets. You'll have to approach the campsite with a small watercraft. Whether you choose a sailboat, a motorboat, or, better yet, a canoe or kayak, is entirely up to you.

Selden Neck comprises four discrete camping areas: Hogback, Springledge, Quarry Knob, and Cedars, listed roughly in order of my personal preference. The first three areas are situated along the banks of the Connecticut River. The main channel runs down the river right next to Selden Neck, so on a busy summer day there will be lots of boat traffic, including some ferry boats and sizable powerboats. Consequently, it can be a bit busy during the day, and there may be some chop on the river and splashing up against the banks of Selden Neck. Secure your boat adequately, or pull your canoe or kayak up onto the shore to keep it from getting bashed around—or worse, from slipping off into the river without you.

The Hogback, Springledge, and Quarry Knob areas are similar, with small, grassy areas upon which to pitch your tent. You'll be fairly close to the riverbanks, and behind the sites a short, steep hill rises in the center of the island. Hogback is the smallest of these areas, with room for 6 campers. Springledge accommodates 8 campers, and Quarry Knob has room for 12.

> *Selden Neck has some of the most spectacular and accessible island camping in New England.*

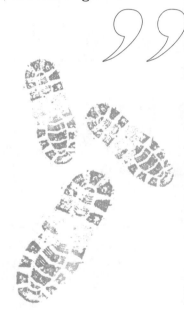

RATINGS

Beauty: ✩ ✩ ✩ ✩
Privacy: ✩ ✩ ✩ ✩ ✩
Spaciousness: ✩ ✩ ✩ ✩ ✩
Quiet: ✩ ✩ ✩ ✩
Security: ✩ ✩ ✩ ✩ ✩
Cleanliness: ✩ ✩ ✩ ✩

KEY INFORMATION

ADDRESS: c/o Gillette Castle
State Park
67 River Rd.
Haddam, CT 06423

OPERATED BY: Connecticut
Department of
Energy and
Environmental
Protection

INFORMATION: 860-526-2336

OPEN: May 1–Sept. 30

SITES: 4 sites accommo-
dating 46 people
total

EACH SITE: Fire pit, pit toilet

ASSIGNMENT: Reservations
required; make
at least 2 weeks
before visit by
mail to the Gillette
Castle State Park
Supervisor (address
above); include full
payment by check
or money order
made out to the
Connecticut state
treasurer

REGISTRATION: Claim your site

FACILITIES: Pit toilets

PARKING: Boats only

FEE: $5 per person,
per night

RESTRICTIONS: *Pets:* Prohibited
Fires: In fire pits
only
Alcohol: At sites only
Vehicles: Boats only
Other: Visitors must
leave by 8 p.m.;
campers must pack
out all trash

You can really immerse yourself in wilderness and solitude here, even though you're camping right on the Connecticut River, which can sometimes feel like the maritime equivalent of an interstate. The small, densely forested camping areas, the way they are set off from each other, and the fact that you're on an island all contribute to the atmosphere of isolation on Selden Neck. This becomes even more apparent toward the end of the day as the river traffic quiets down.

The Cedars area attracts a lot of day use, as it's tucked into a corner of Selden Creek off the main branch of the river. If the weather or winds are rough, this would be a good choice because the small beach where you arrive is more protected. It's also a good choice if you happen to be camping with a larger group: this area of Selden Neck can accommodate up to 20 people.

The nearest boat ramp is the Deep River public boat launch, right across the river from Selden Creek and the island on which the campground is located. It's a fairly short paddle in a canoe or kayak, and a snap in a small motorboat or sailboat. The only trouble is parking at the boat launch—it's reserved only for Deep River residents who have purchased a sticker. Get dropped off or park just outside the boat-launch parking area, if there's room.

Keep the following in mind as you prepare for your trip: You are traveling to an island to camp. There are no stores on this island. You need to bring everything with you—all your food, water, and camping supplies. Running out to a store because you forgot batteries or hot dogs is not impossible, but it's not going to be easy. The flip side of that coin is that you must also pack out everything you've used as well as any trash you've generated. The camping areas have pit toilets, but there aren't any garbage cans. Live by the pack-it-in, pack-it-out mantra.

When kayak-camping (or taking canoes or other small boats), cook something you can freeze in Tupperware. By dinnertime, your meal will have mostly defrosted. Then just heat it up and dinner is served.

Once you make landfall and set up your camp, you'll probably want to take off in your boat to do a little exploring. Selden Creek, which winds its way

MAP

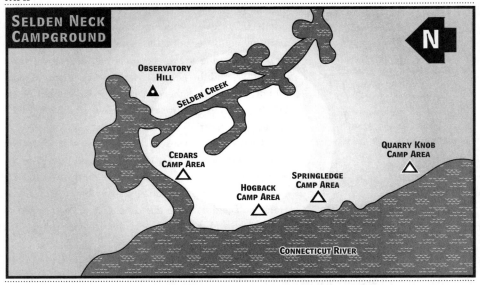

SELDEN NECK CAMPGROUND

N

OBSERVATORY HILL
△

SELDEN CREEK

CEDARS CAMP AREA
△

SPRINGLEDGE CAMP AREA
△

QUARRY KNOB CAMP AREA
△

HOGBACK CAMP AREA
△

CONNECTICUT RIVER

around Selden Neck Island, is an absolutely delightful area to paddle. The water is often as still as glass, even on days when the wind has churned the main channel of the river into a swirling froth. The creek winds casually around through swampy marsh and overhanging trees, past some cliffs and the forested hills of the mainland. At times it feels like you're paddling through a bayou, at others through a northern fjord, but it always feels like you're a million miles from anyone.

One important (unexpected) caveat: beware of the swans. They are beautiful birds, there are plenty of them, and they are fiercely territorial. I've been charged by swans on three separate occasions while paddling through Selden Creek. It's kind of ridiculous from a human's point of view. I was in a 17-foot-long, bright-yellow kayak. Still, this stubborn, ornery swan charged me broadside.

Besides the fact that it's always best to view wildlife from a respectful distance so that your presence has as little effect on their behavior as possible, it pays to be mindful of how close you are to the swans. If you get too close and they attack, they could poke a hole in a fiberglass canoe or kayak or, worse yet, break your arm

GETTING THERE

To get to the Deep River boat launch, take Exit 4 off CT 9. Follow CT 154 into Deep River. Turn right at the four-way intersection downtown (CT 80 heads off to the left). Follow this road to the boat launch.

GPS COORDINATES

N41° 24.120855'
W72° 25.140524'

or wrist. Those long, slender necks are solid muscle. If a swan starts posturing, appears agitated, or tucks its wings up into attack mode so it looks like a Romulan Warbird (for you Trekkies out there), simply continue on your way and it'll eventually leave you alone to enjoy the otherwise peaceful and pristine solitude of Selden Creek.

With a campfire crackling in the fire pit, a belly full of dinner, and a warm glow on your face from spending the day on and around the water, sit back at your campsite and admire the river as it slows down for the night. Looking west across the river from the Hogback, Springledge, and Quarry Knob sites, you'll have a beautiful view of the opposite riverbank and the top of Gillette Castle. When the weather is right, you're at one of the best spots in Connecticut from which to admire the sunset.

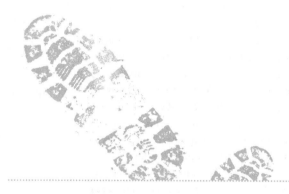

RHODE ISLAND

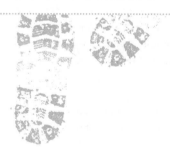

59
FORT GETTY
RECREATION AREA

FORT GETTY RECREATION AREA will appeal to history buffs and anyone wanting to combine a little paddling or beachcombing with their camping experience. It's also a perfect spot for capturing some island-camping mystique without actually loading up a boat, canoe, or kayak and rowing off across the water. Set on a windswept bluff near the southern tip of Conanicut Island, in the middle of Narragansett Bay, this is a beautiful oceanside campground. Even though it's on an island, rest assured you can get there by car. What it lacks in privacy and distance from the nearby flotilla of RVs, it makes up for in salty sea breezes, sunrises and sunsets to die for, rocky beachfronts worth hours of exploring, and a fantastic place to drop a kayak or a hook in the water.

The two modestly sized tent-camping areas are set off as much as possible from where the RVs roam. I say "as much as possible" because there isn't a whole lot of room within the campground proper. The scenery and setting compensate nicely for the forest density, though. Here's a hint: once you've found your campsite, set up your tent so the opening faces the bay. That way, when you wake up, your first views will be of the sun rising over the water.

As you drive into the park, the long access road leading into the campground passes a couple of residences, so it feels like you're heading up someone's driveway, but keep on—this road does indeed lead to Fort Getty Recreation Area. You'll come to a pay station in the middle of the road. Check in here, then keep cruising. The road winds around to the right and the campground is ahead on the left, toward the end of the peninsula.

As you drive in, you'll pass the Fox Hill Salt Marsh on your right. This is a great place to walk around or to just find a cozy spot to take in the scenery. If you're into birding, you'll particularly enjoy training your eyes and binoculars on the various shorebirds found here. You'll

> *Fort Getty Recreation Area's campground is fairly wide open, but the panoramic vistas of Narragansett Bay and the sea breezes can't be beat.*

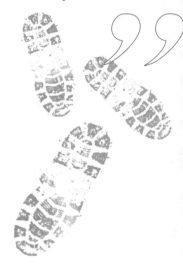

RATINGS

Beauty: ✩ ✩ ✩ ✩
Privacy: ✩ ✩
Spaciousness: ✩ ✩ ✩
Quiet: ✩ ✩ ✩
Security: ✩ ✩ ✩ ✩
Cleanliness: ✩ ✩ ✩ ✩

KEY INFORMATION

ADDRESS: P.O. Box 377
Jamestown, RI
02835

OPERATED BY: Town of
Jamestown

INFORMATION: 401-423-7211

OPEN: Mid-May–early Oct.

SITES: 22 tent-only sites,
105 RV sites

EACH SITE: Fire ring

ASSIGNMENT: First-come,
first-served

REGISTRATION: At ranger station

FACILITIES: Flush toilets, showers, water spigots,
pay phones, boat
launch, fishing
dock, horseshoe
pits, saltwater
beach

PARKING: Near sites; additional parking at
day-use area

FEE: $25

RESTRICTIONS: *Pets:* Dogs on
leash only
Fires: In fire rings
only
Alcohol: At sites only
Vehicles: 1 per site

quickly realize that the campground at Fort Getty doesn't embody the forest-bound sense of solitude you'll find in most other New England campgrounds, but the water-front setting can't be beat. The tent-only area, toward the top of the small hill off to the left as you reach the campsites, includes sites 1 through 15. These sites are all very open and fairly tightly packed, but parking for them is along the periphery, so the site cluster feels like a little tent village.

Right next to the camping area is a big open field; it's a tremendous spot for picnicking, kite-flying, Frisbee-throwing—you name it. There's also a sand-volleyball pit nearby. This space for casual play and hanging out rein-forces the laid-back island mentality that predominates at Fort Getty.

The second batch of tent sites is across the main road from the salt marsh. After you pass the gate house, there will be a road off to the left that leads to tent sites 16 through 22. These are set well off on their own and are farther from the RV area, so they are much more quiet. However, they lack the waterfront location of sites 1 through 15.

Camping with little kids? The rocky beaches sur-rounding the park offer endless hours of rock-hopping and beachcombing. Some of the cliffs and larger rocks are a bit steep, so you'll have to keep a sharp eye on the younger ones, but I can guarantee your kids will be tuck-ered out after a day spent prowling these rocky shores.

For the historically minded, a couple of bunkers remain from when Fort Getty was an ammunition depot during World War II. These are also cool little spots in which older kids enjoy playing.

Conanicut Island is surrounded by several other small islands. In a place like this, the environment is cap-tivating regardless of the weather. It's brilliant on bright, sunny days, and cool and refreshing when the mainland is sweltering. The stars at night are crystal-clear, and you'll see deeper into the universe since there isn't much in the way of light pollution out here. In a fog or light rain, the islands poking in and out of the mist give the place a sense of mystery, as if you'd almost expect to see a pirate ship emerging to bury its sailors' stolen treasures on one of the islands.

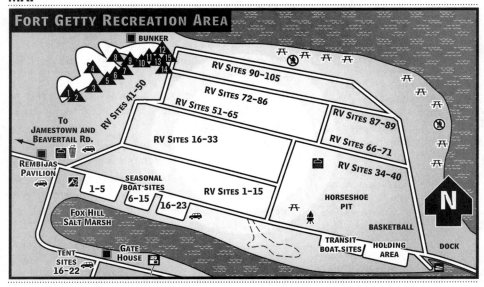

FORT GETTY RECREATION AREA

BUNKER

RV SITES 90-105

RV SITES 72-86

RV SITES 51-65

RV SITES 41-50

RV SITES 87-89

RV SITES 66-71

To
JAMESTOWN AND
BEAVERTAIL RD.

RV SITES 16-33

RV SITES 34-40

REMBIJAS
PAVILION

1-5

SEASONAL
BOAT SITES

6-15   16-23

RV SITES 1-15

HORSESHOE
PIT

FOX HILL
SALT MARSH

N

BASKETBALL

TRANSIT-
BOAT SITES

HOLDING
AREA

DOCK

TENT
SITES
16-22

GATE
HOUSE

If you're planning a family reunion, wedding reception, or some other big bash, you can reserve the Lt. Col. John C. Rembijas Pavilion for such functions. This is off to the left of the campground, open field, and volleyball pit; call for more information on reserving the space.

Fort Getty Recreation Area is scenic and centrally located: a perfect base camp for fishing (for information on fishing licenses, see Appendix C, page 232), paddling, scuba diving, and beachcombing. It's also an amazing place to fly a kite. Charlie Brown would have loved it—steady winds and few kite-eating trees to be found. Those winds also make Fort Getty Recreation Area the place to be on steamy summer afternoons. While folks camping deep in the forest are sweating bullets and swatting away bugs, you'll have a strong, cool breeze keeping your temperature down and the bugs at bay.

GETTING THERE

Take North Main Road in Jamestown to the south (toward Beavertail State Park). This road will cross Narragansett Road and turn into Southwest Avenue, then Beavertail Road. This winds around a sandy beach to the left, and the entrance for the campground is on the right.

GPS COORDINATES

N41° 29.275296'
W71° 23.865488'

60
GEORGE WASHINGTON MANAGEMENT AREA

> *The entire George Washington Management Area is a lush, dense forest that is quite accessible yet has a pleasant, remote feel.*

YOU'LL BE TEMPTED to check your map as you drive into the campground at the George Washington Management Area. Did you somehow take a wrong turn and end up in Vermont or New Hampshire? Nope, this is indeed Rhode Island, but it's far from the windswept beaches, sandy soil, and short, scrubby pines and beach roses you might expect of Rhode Island topography. As soon as you enter the campground, you are enshrouded by a canopy of conifers. The tangy pine and balsam scents, mixed in with earthy wisps of wood smoke, make for quite a welcome.

The entire George Washington Management Area and the contiguous Pulaski Memorial State Forest are both densely wooded areas with a gently rolling forest floor. The area is free of really steep hills, uneven terrain, and heavy undergrowth. This makes for many nice places to pitch a tent. Stop to pay your fee at the ranger station as you drive into the campground, and you're ready to go.

The campground wraps around the shores of Bowdish Reservoir. Down by the beach area is a beautiful stone recreation hall built by the Civilian Conservation Corps (CCC). A plaque in front of the building honors the members of the CCC who built the hall. The beach is the perfect spot to go for a quick swim, to spend the day with the kids, or to kick back on a blanket and read a book. You could also drop a hook or a paddle in the water (or both!) if you're so inclined.

Sites 26, 27, and 28 are quite spacious and close to the lake. These are some of the best camping spots in the management area. The loop with sites 36 through 45 has other good spots in which to pitch your tent. The sites within this loop are a bit smaller than some of those along the main campground road, but they're nestled within a dense pine grove and fairly close to the lake—both attractive aspects. This loop is the first left off the main road once you're in the campground.

RATINGS

Beauty: ✪ ✪ ✪ ✪
Privacy: ✪ ✪ ✪ ✪
Spaciousness: ✪ ✪ ✪ ✪
Quiet: ✪ ✪ ✪ ✪
Security: ✪ ✪ ✪ ✪
Cleanliness: ✪ ✪ ✪ ✪

Farther down the road, sites 8, 9, 12 and 13 are well worth investigating. The forest becomes denser on this end of the campground.

Follow the main campground road past all these sites and past the loop for Shelter 1 off to the left, and you'll be heading off into the rest of the George Washington Management Area. This is a great place to explore when it's time for a hike or bike ride.

The entire campground has plenty of space and forest for everyone. If you've come with a large group or you have several members of your group who would rather not sleep on the ground, check out one of the two Appalachian Mountain Club–type lean-to shelters. Each has a wood floor and is open on one side. If you're going for one of the shelters, try to secure Shelter 1. It's up on a small rise at the end of its own loop, offering some privacy. It's at the far end of the campground road, and right on the border between the campground and the rest of the expansive management area. Shelter 2 is also in a nice spot, quite separate from the rest of the campground at the end of a short road leading off to the right from the main campground road.

A restriction worth noting: possession of alcoholic beverages is grounds for expulsion. The campground management must have had some problems with rowdy revelers in the past, as they seem quite serious about this rule, which is clearly stated in several spots in the campground literature. If you like to kick back with a beer or a glass of wine after dinner, try a cup of tea instead.

Another point to ponder is the wildlife: let it remain wild. Don't feed or otherwise tempt animals by leaving food or dirty dishes around your campsite. The George Washington Management Area campground is wild and scenic, but it's also very accessible. Once otherwise-wild animals become acclimated to human's presence, they often have to be relocated or exterminated—and you don't want to be responsible for that. Plus, there are general safety considerations: raccoons can carry rabies, so report any incidences of raccoon or other animal bites or scrapes. It's also a good idea to report any strange or aggressive animal behavior.

At 3,500 acres, the George Washington Management Area is big enough to be a one-stop-shopping type

ADDRESS: 2185 Putnam Pike Chepachet, RI 02814

OPERATED BY: Rhode Island Department of Environmental Management–Division of Forest Environment

INFORMATION: 401-568-6700 or 401-568-2085

OPEN: Mid-April–late Oct.

SITES: 45 sites, 2 shelters, 5 group sites

EACH SITE: Fire ring

ASSIGNMENT: At registration when you pay for permit or by reservation at reserve america.com

REGISTRATION: At pay station near campground entrance or office in recreation hall

FACILITIES: Toilets, water spigots, boat launch

PARKING: At campsites; extra parking available at recreation hall and Shelter 1

FEE: Rhode Island residents, $14; nonresidents, $20; shelters, $35

RESTRICTIONS: *Pets:* Not allowed
Fires: In fire rings
Alcohol: Not allowed
Vehicles: 1 per site; second vehicle for $4 (Rhode Island residents) or $6 (nonresidents)
Other: 14-day maximum stay; visitors must leave by 10 p.m.; quiet hours 10 p.m.–7 a.m.

MAP

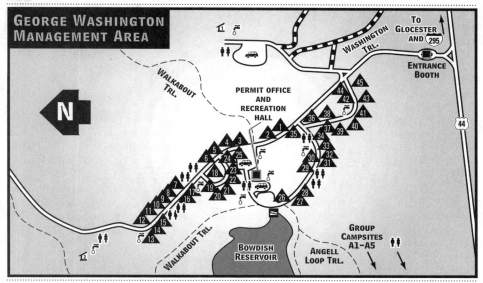

GETTING THERE

From I-295, follow US 44 West through Greenville and Chepachet into Glocester. Keep an eye out for the campground sign, on the right.

GPS COORDINATES

N41° 55.186164'
W71° 45.300508'

of place for outdoor adventure. Bowdish Reservoir is right there for swimming, fishing, and paddling. The network of trails winding through the George Washington Management Area and Pulaski Memorial State Forest will keep the hikers and mountain bikers in your group busy for days.

The Walkabout Trail, marked by orange and red dots, is an 8-mile hike that passes by Wilbur Pond, a beautiful hemlock grove, and some wetlands. The trail leads right out of the campground. There are several alternate-trail options along the way for those who don't want to go the full 8 miles. The blue-dot-marked cutoff makes it a 2-mile hike, and the red-dot-marked cutoff makes it a 6-mile hike.

A tiny sign at the apex of the roof on the backside of the ranger station sums up the friendly nature of the George Washington Management Area. Look closely, drive slowly, look up, and you'll see it as you're leaving—HAVE A NICE DAY, with the classic yellow smiley face.

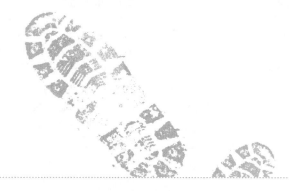

APPENDIXES

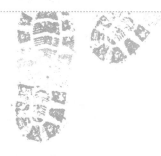

APPENDIX A: CAMPING-EQUIPMENT CHECKLIST

I keep a plastic storage container full of the essentials for car camping—except for the large and bulky items that won't fit—so they're ready to go when I am. I make a last-minute check of the inventory, resupply anything that's low or missing, and take off!

COOKING UTENSILS

Aluminum foil

Bottle opener

Bottles of salt, pepper, spices, sugar, cooking oil, and maple syrup in waterproof, spillproof containers

Can opener

Corkscrew

Cups, plastic or tin

Dish soap (biodegradable), sponge, and towel

Flatware

Food of your choice

Frying pan

Fuel for stove

Matches in waterproof container

Plates

Pocketknife or multitool

Pot with lid

Spatula

Stove

Wooden spoon

FIRST-AID KIT

Antibiotic cream

Adhesive bandages

Diphenhydramine (Benadryl)

Gauze pads

Ibuprofen or aspirin

Insect repellent

Lip balm

Moleskin/Spenco 2nd Skin

Snakebite kit

Sunscreen

Tape and waterproof adhesive

SLEEPING GEAR

Pillow

Sleeping bag

Sleeping pad, inflatable or insulated

Tent with ground tarp and rainfly

MISCELLANEOUS

Bath soap (biodegradable), washcloth, towel

Camp chair

Candles

Cooler

Deck of cards

Duct tape

Fire starter

Flashlight or headlamp with fresh batteries

Foul-weather clothing

Lantern

Paper towels

Plastic zip-top bags

Sunglasses

Toilet paper

Water bottle

Wool or fleece blanket

OPTIONAL

Barbecue grill

Binoculars

Field guides on bird, plant, and wildlife identification

Fishing rod and tackle

GPS unit or compass

Hatchet

Kayak and paddling gear

Maps (road, topographic, trail, and so on)

Mountain bike and gear

APPENDIX B: SOURCES OF INFORMATION

MAINE

MAINE BUREAU OF PARKS AND LANDS
22 State House Station
18 Elkins Lane (AMHI Campus)
Augusta, ME 04333
207-287-3821
maine.gov/doc/parks

NATIONAL PARK SERVICE
Acadia National Park
P.O. Box 177
ME 233, McFarland Hill
Bar Harbor, ME 04609
207-288-3338
nps.gov/acad

NEW HAMPSHIRE

NEW HAMPSHIRE DEPARTMENT OF RESOURCES AND ECONOMIC DEVELOPMENT
Division of Parks and Recreation
172 Pembroke Road
P.O. Box 1856
Concord, NH 03302-1856
603-271-3556
nhstateparks.org

UNITED STATES DEPARTMENT OF AGRICULTURE–U.S. FOREST SERVICE
White Mountain National Forest
71 White Mountain Drive
Campton, NH 03223
603-536-6100
fs.usda.gov/whitemountain

VERMONT

VERMONT DEPARTMENT OF FORESTS, PARKS, & RECREATION
103 S. Main St.
Waterbury, VT 05671-0603
802-241-3655
vtstateparks.com

UNITED STATES DEPARTMENT OF AGRICULTURE–U.S. FOREST SERVICE
Green Mountain National Forest
231 N. Main St.
Rutland, VT 05701
802-747-6700
fs.usda.gov/greenmountain

MASSACHUSETTS

MASSACHUSETTS DEPARTMENT OF CONSERVATION AND RECREATION
251 Causeway St.
Boston, MA 02114-2104
617-626-1250
mass.gov/dcr

CONNECTICUT

CONNECTICUT DEPARTMENT OF ENERGY AND ENVIRONMENTAL PROTECTION
79 Elm St.
Hartford, CT 06106-5127
860-424-3000
ct.gov/dep

RHODE ISLAND

RHODE ISLAND DEPARTMENT OF ENVIRONMENTAL MANAGEMENT
2321 Hartford Ave.
Johnston, RI 02919
401-222-2632
riparks.com

APPENDIX C
FISHING-LICENSE
INFORMATION

Note: Rates, unless indicated, are for annual passes for individuals ages 16 and older (younger kids don't need them). These fees are likely to change every year, so call to inquire about current rates and/or hunting licenses.

MAINE
207-287-8000
$25 for residents; $64 for nonresidents; $23 for a three-day pass

NEW HAMPSHIRE
603-271-3211
$35 for residents; $53 for nonresidents; $28 for a three-day pass

VERMONT
802-241-3700
$22 for residents; $45 for nonresidents; $22 for a three-day pass

MASSACHUSETTS
508-389-6300
$27.50 for residents; $37.50 for nonresidents; $11.50 for ages 15–17; $23.50 for a three-day pass

CONNECTICUT
860-424-3105
$28 for residents; $55 for nonresidents; $22 for a three-day pass

RHODE ISLAND
401-423-1920
$18 for residents; $35 for nonresidents; $16 for a three-day pass

INDEX

A

Acadia National Park (ME), 16, 40, 41, 50, 231
AMC (Appalachian Mountain Club), 9
AMC Outdoors magazine, 9
animal, plant hazards, 6, 7
Appalachian Mountain Club (AMC), 9
Appalachian Trail, 13, 115, 126, 129, 147, 160, 162

B

Bald Mountain (ME), 37, 49
Ball Mountain Dam (VT), 141
Baxter, Percival, 12
Baxter State Park (ME), 12–15
Bear Brook State Park (NH), 60–62
Beartown State Forest (MA), 160–162
Beauty (campground profile), 2–3
Benedict Pond (MA), 160, 161
Big Coolidge Mountain (NH), 87
Big Rock Campground (NH), 63–65
Black Mountain (NH), 87
Blackberry Crossing Campground (NH), 66–68
Blackwoods Campground (ME), 16–18
Blueberry Mountain (ME), 37
Boston Harbor Islands (MA), 163–167
Bowdish Reservoir (RI), 225, 227
Bradbury Mountain State Park (ME), 19–21
Branbury State Park (VT), 112–114
Bumpkin Island (MA), 165, 167
Burrage Children's Hospital (MA), 165

C

Cadillac Mountain (ME), 17, 18
campgrounds
  See also specific campground
  in Connecticut, 203–219
  in Maine, 11–57
  in Massachusetts, 159–201
  in New Hampshire, 59–109
  profiles generally, 2–4
  rating system, 2–3
  reserving sites, 6
  in Rhode Island, 221–227
  venturing away from, 8
  in Vermont, 111–158
camping
  animal, plant hazards, 6
  canoe and kayak, 4–5
  equipment checklist, 230
  etiquette, 7–8
Cannon Mountain (NH), 92
canoe camping, 4–5
Cathedral Ledge (NH), 63
Champney Falls (NH), 91
Chapman Falls (CT), 204, 205
Chase Mountain (CT), 211
checklist for camping equipment, 230
Childs River (MA), 195
Chittenden Brook Recreation Area (VT), 115–117
Civilian Conservation Corps, 66
Clarksburg State Park (MA), 168–170
Cleanliness (campground profile), 3
Cliff Pond, Nickerson State Park (MA), 181
clothing, 6–7
Cobble Mountain (CT), 212
Cobscook Bay State Park (ME), 22–25
Cold River (MA), 174, 175
Conanicut Island (RI), 222–223
Connecticut
  featured campgrounds, 203–219
  fishing-license information, 232
  sources of information, 231
Connecticut River, 216, 217
Coolidge, Pres. Calvin, 118

P

Passaconaway Campground (NH), 96–98
Pawtuckaway Lake (NH), 99–100
Pawtuckaway State Park (NH), 99–103
Peabody River (NH), 77
Peaks-Kenny State Park (ME), 43–45
Pemigewasset River (NH), 87, 93
Penobscot Bay (NH), 56–57
permits, 7
Perseid meteor showers, 66
Pillsbury State Park (NH), 104–106
plant, animal, hazards, 6, 7
poison ivy, oak, sumac, 6
Potash Knob (NH), 87
Privacy (campground profile), 3
profiles, campground, 2–4
Pulaski Memorial State Forest (RI), 225, 227

Q

Quechee State Park (VT), 149–152
Quiet (campground profile), 3

R

Rangeley Lake State Park (ME), 46–49
rating system for campgrounds, 2–3
reserving sites, 6
Rhode Island
    featured campgrounds, 221–227
    fishing-license information, 232
    sources of information, 231
Rocky Gorge (NH), 67
Roosevelt, Pres. Franklin D., 67

S

Saco River (NH), 72, 73, 75
Savoy Mountain State Forest (MA), 184–186
Seawall Campground (ME), 50–53
Sebago Lake (ME), 48
Sebec Lake (ME), 43
security
    animal, plant hazards, 6
    first-aid-kit contents, 5, 205, 230
Security (campground profile), 3

Selden Neck Campground (CT), 216–219
Shawme-Crowell State Forest (MA), 187–190
Smugglers Notch State Park (VT), 153–155
Somerset Reservoir (VT), 130
Somes Sound (ME), 40, 41
Spaciousness (campground profile), 3
star-rating system for campgrounds, 2–3
Stowe Mountain Resort (VT), 153
streams, crossing, 8
sumac, poison, 6
Swift River (NH), 67, 69, 89, 91

T

tents, 7
testing your canoe or kayak, 4–5
this book, this revision, 1–2
Three Sisters (NH), 91
ticks, 6, 205
Tolland State Forest (MA), 191–194
trash, 7
Tuckerman Ravine (NH), 78
Tumbledown Mountain (ME), 37
Turner Mountain (ME), 13

U

Underhill State Park (VT), 156–158

V

venturing away from campgrounds, 8
Vermont
    featured campgrounds, 111–158
    fishing-license information, 232
    sources of information, 231

W

Waquoit Bay National Estuarine Research
    Reserve (MA), 195–197
Warren Island State Park (ME), 54–57
Washburn Island (MA), 195, 196
water
    canoe/kayak camping, 4–5
    drinking, 8

ABOUT THE AUTHOR

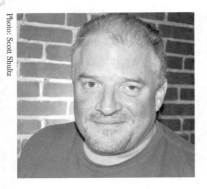

Photo: Scott Shultz

LAFE LOW, a lifelong New Englander, spends nearly all his free time outside—skiing, camping, skiing, mountain biking, skiing, kayaking, and skiing . . . you get the picture. He first started camping in grade school, when he and his best friend, Dan Quagliaroli, would head off into the woods of southern Connecticut most Saturday afternoons with lofty ideals, indomitable spirit, and ridiculously heavy backpacks.

After earning a bachelor of arts degree in journalism from Keene State College in 1984, Lafe went to work in the magazine world. After working for a variety of technology publications, he launched his own magazine, *Explore New England,* in 1995. This was the crossroads of his personal and professional passions. After *Explore New England,* he went on to be the editor of *Outdoor Adventure* and an editor for the Globe Pequot Press. He is now the editor-in-chief of a technology website. *The Best in Tent Camping: New England* is his first book, but not his last. He lives in the Boston area.

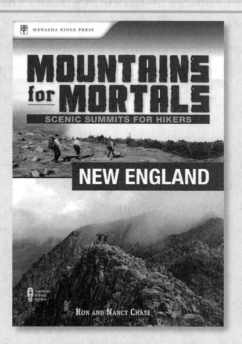
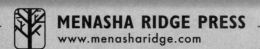

DEAR CUSTOMERS AND FRIENDS,

SUPPORTING YOUR INTEREST IN OUTDOOR ADVENTURE, travel, and an active lifestyle is central to our operations, from the authors we choose to the locations we detail to the way we design our books. Menasha Ridge Press was incorporated in 1982 by a group of veteran outdoorsmen and professional outfitters. For many years now, we've specialized in creating books that benefit the outdoors enthusiast.

Almost immediately, Menasha Ridge Press earned a reputation for revolutionizing outdoors- and travel-guidebook publishing. For such activities as canoeing, kayaking, hiking, backpacking, and mountain biking, we established new standards of quality that transformed the whole genre, resulting in outdoor-recreation guides of great sophistication and solid content. Menasha Ridge continues to be outdoor publishing's greatest innovator.

The folks at Menasha Ridge Press are as at home on a white-water river or mountain trail as they are editing a manuscript. The books we build for you are the best they can be, because we're responding to your needs. Plus, we use and depend on them ourselves.

We look forward to seeing you on the river or the trail. If you'd like to contact us directly, join in at www.trekalong.com or visit us at www.menasharidge.com. We thank you for your interest in our books and the natural world around us all.

SAFE TRAVELS,

BOB SEHLINGER
PUBLISHER